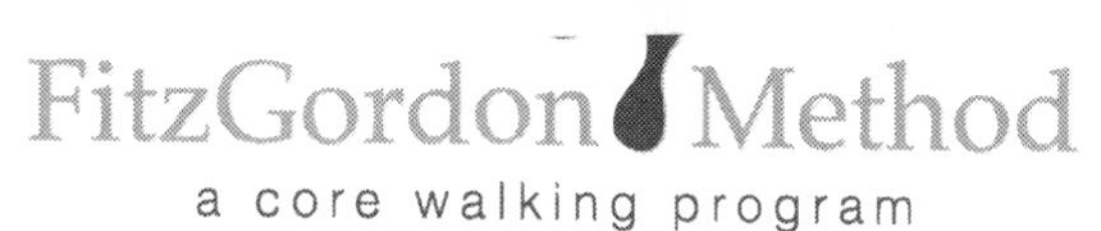

The Exercises of the FitzGordon Method

The Core Collection

Jonathan FitzGordon

www.FitzGordonMethod.com

Other books in this series:

Psoas Release Party!

Sciatica / Piriformis Syndrome

An Introduction to The Spine

www.FitzGordonMethod.com

TABLE OF CONTENTS

I. INTRODUCTION

This book is a basic collection of exercises that we offer to clients of the FitzGordon Method Core Walking Program. Any one who walks in our door will receive a series of exercises meant to create a workout tailored for them specifically. We all need to work on different parts of their body to create a balanced whole and no two people are the same. At the FitzGordon Method we analyze our clients to help them rebuild their bodies in a conscious and specific way.

While we work with all of these exercises and more, the idea is to only do the exercises you need to bring balance to a certain part of your body. You should test your ability in all of these exercises and, as long as you are doing them correctly, focus only on the ones that seem more difficult.

The work is a search for ease in the body and ease in the mind. Once an exercise becomes easy to do you might do it occassionally for maintenance. However, continually focus on the muscle groups that don't work as well as others and maintain the discipline required to develop a balanced body.

This is not intended to be an instruction manual. We highly recommend that anyone interested in this work sign up to take our Walking Program.

You will need the following to do the exercises:

- Mat
- Belt
- Two blocks
- Tennis Ball
- Squishy Ball

II . The Core

1. Pelvic Floor

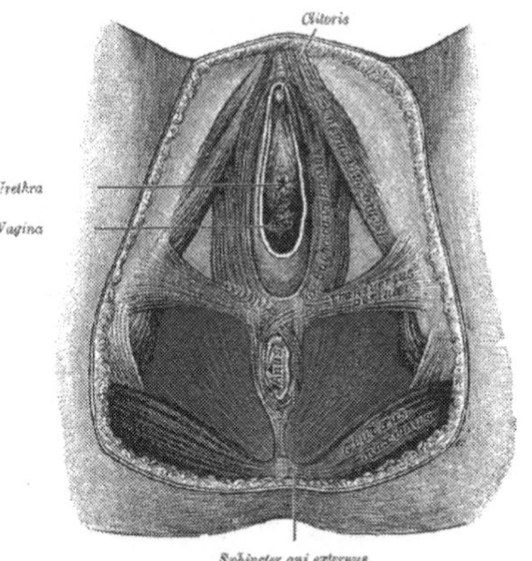

The pelvic floor is a large sling, or hammock, of muscles stretching from side to side across the floor of the pelvis. It is attached to your pubic bone in front, and to the coccyx (the tail end of the spine) in back. Make sure not to use your butt muscles in any of these exercises.

Doing these exercises correctly will help you find the correct placement of the pelvis which is key to all of the work we are trying to do.

When you tone or lift the pelvic floor the energetic quality should be a free lift up the central channel of the spine. If your pelvis is tucked under it is likely that your pubic bone will interrupt or stop the lift of the pelvic floor. Likewise, if your pelvis is rotated too far backwards you might feel that the sacrum or the back of the pelvis stops the upward flow of the pelvis floor. You know your pelvis is in the right place if the

lift of the pelvic floor goes straight up the front of the spine.

There are three layers to the pelvic floor. You are trying to find the top layer, just slightly above holding in your pee (it can be very subtle).

- Tone your pelvic floor muscles, hold for a count of five. Do in sets of ten.
- Tone and lift your pelvic floor slowly, trying to stop and start as you go up, like an elevator stopping on several floors.
- If that seems easy enough try doing the opposite, lifting the pelvic floor, holding it at the top and lowering it incrementally.
- Practice quick contractions, drawing in the pelvic floor and holding for just one second before releasing the muscles. Do these in a steady manner aiming for a strong contraction each time building up to a count of fifty.

2. Feet 3 Inches off the Floor

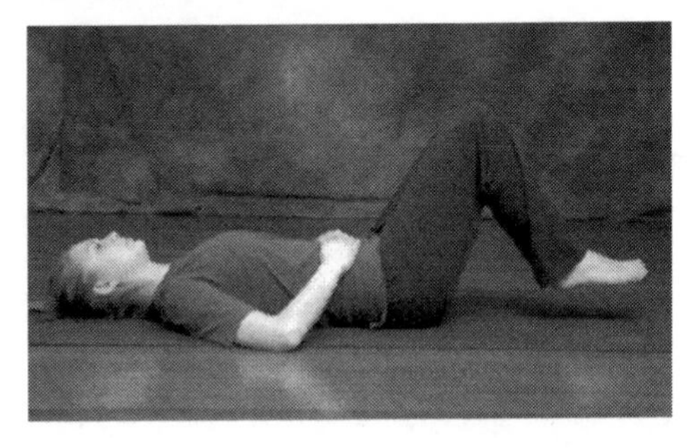

This exercise works the deep low belly muscle called the transverse abdominus. First, we'll show how this muscle works and then how another abdominal muscle, the rectus abdominus, works.

- Lie on your back on your mat. Bend your knees so that your feet are resting on the floor beneath your knees. Bring your hands onto the lower belly. Inhale and exhale. Inhale again and exhale but this time push the exhale at the end and see if you feel your navel move down to the spine and the muscle engagement seems as if it wraps from the back to the front. Let that go.
- Now lift your head and shoulders and look at your knees. Here you should feel the belly push up into the fingers. Let the head release.

The first muscle that we engaged was called the transverse abdominis, a muscle that supports the lower back and wraps from the back to the front. The second muscle we engaged is called the rectus abdominis and connects the pelvis to the rib cage and moves in a direction straight up and down. We're going to try to isolate and engage only the deeper transverse muscle.

- Lift your right foot three inches off the floor and try to stabilize the spine as you lift the left foot three inches to meet it. Did the spine move up and the belly push up? Or did the spine actually stabilize and stay still? Release your feet. The goal is to keep the trunk stable.
- Lift the left foot three inches off the floor and lift the right foot three inches to meet it. Feel if the two sides were different.
- When lifting the feet without any movement in the belly or the spine becomes effortless and you can sustain it easily, bring the feet up to the height of the knees and parallel to the floor.
- When this becomes easy extend your knees forward two or three inches.

3. Core Twist (Internal and external Oblique)

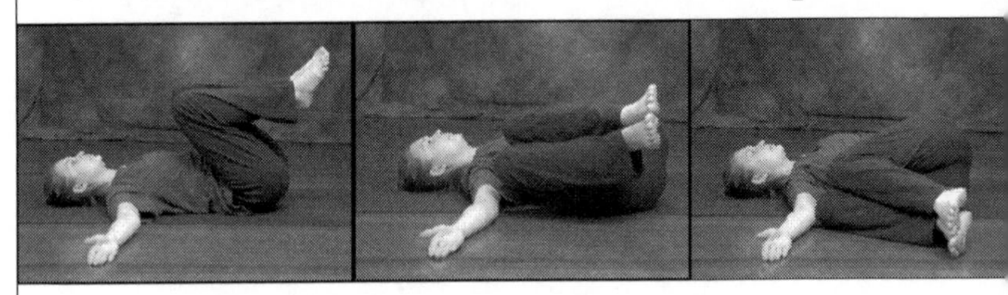

This is a mainstay pose used to work the abdominal muscles known as the internal and external obliques. There is a lot going on in this pose. The inner thighs should stay glued together and the shoulders are resisting the urge to pull off the floor as the legs go over to the opposite side.

- Lie down on your back. Bring your arms out to the side with the wrists at the height of the shoulders, like the letter T. Turn your palms up towards the ceiling.
- Draw your knees up into your chest.
- Attempting to move the knees up slowly, bring your knees over towards the right inner elbow.
- Looking straight up the whole time, keep the legs together and slowly come back up to the center.
- In slow motion, move the knees to the left, again drawing them up towards the elbow.

- Coming back up to the center, keep squeezing the legs together and bring the knees up towards the nose.
- To go deeper in this exercise, come over to the right and stop about two-thirds of the way down. Stop, hold, and squeeze the legs together and release the left side of the rib cage down towards the floor. Come back up to center slowly. Move to the left on an angle as slowly as you can, stop two-thirds of the way, hover and at the same time reach the right side of the rib cage down towards the floor.
- To go deeper still, the full pose is done with straight legs. The difficulty in this advanced version is keeping the legs straight, together, and moving up on an angle towards the finger tips. If the legs can't move on an angle towards the fingers you should only do this with the knees bent.

4. Block Between the Thighs on the Floor

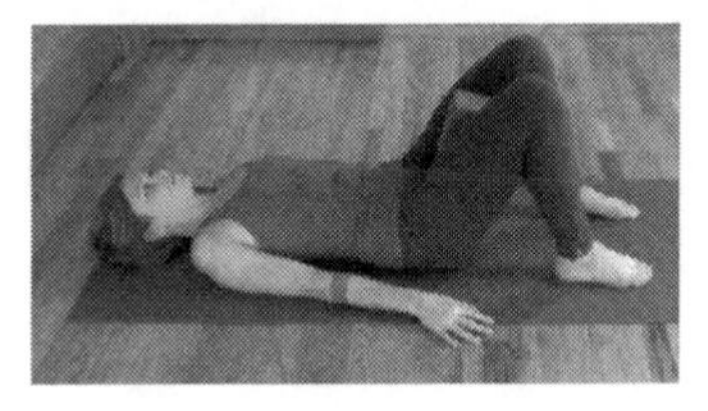

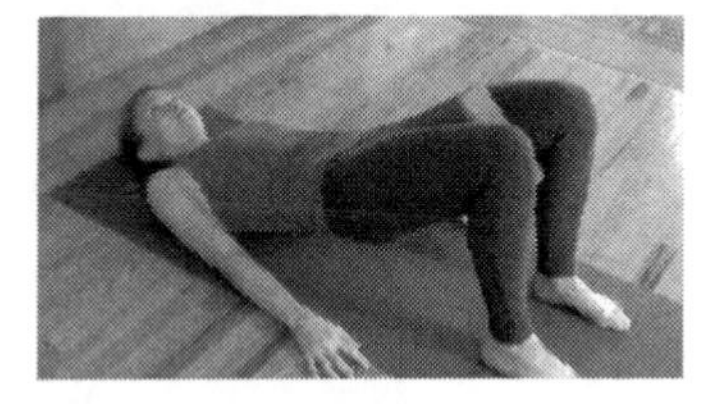

- Lay on your back with the knees bent and your feet flat on the floor.
- Place a block between your inner thighs. Engage and isolate the inner thigh muscles against the block. Use the quadriceps and outer thighs as little as possible.
- Don't grip your buttocks.
- Lift the hips up and continue to squeeze the block, drawing the low belly in to stabilize the spine.
- Hold for a count of 10 breaths. Try to hold longer as you feel stronger. Hold for less if you need to. See if you can build up staying for three minutes.

5. Boat

This classic yoga pose is another way to work the core. The advanced version brings the psoas in and out of engagement.

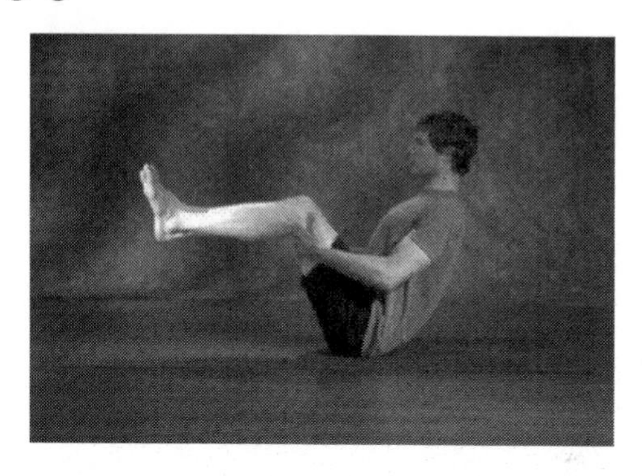

- Sit on the floor with your knees bent and the feet flat. Take hold of the back of your thighs and bring the feet up off the floor. That might be enough, or you might release the hands along side the knees.

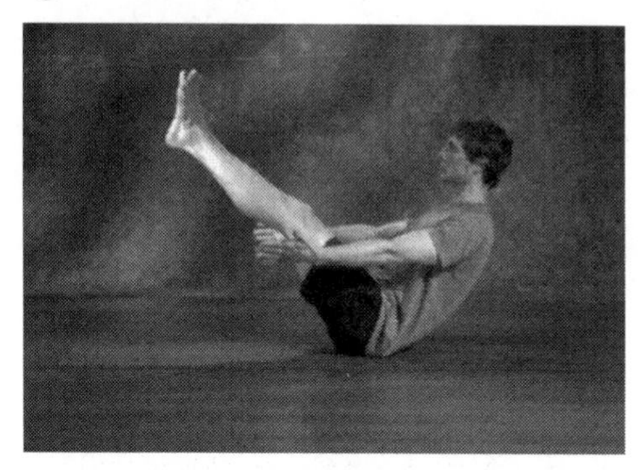

- If possible you can straighten the legs trying to keep the legs and trunk 60 degrees off of the floor. Keep the arms alongside the knees.

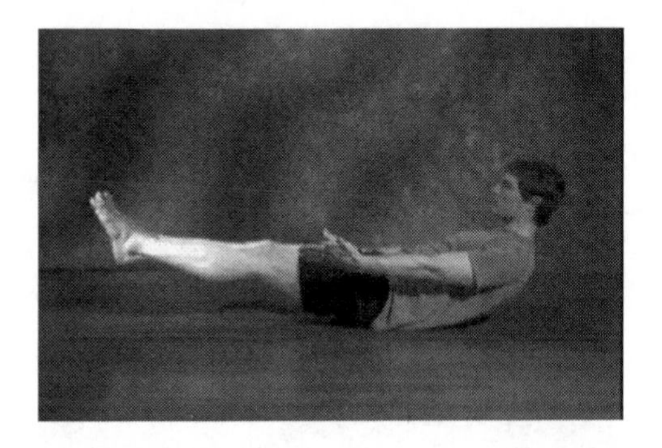

- As this gets easier, lean both the legs and the torso back to about 30 degrees. The back should round a bit and the work of the core should be stronger.
- Try to pull yourself back up to the original position. Repeat five times.

6. Knees One Inch off the Floor

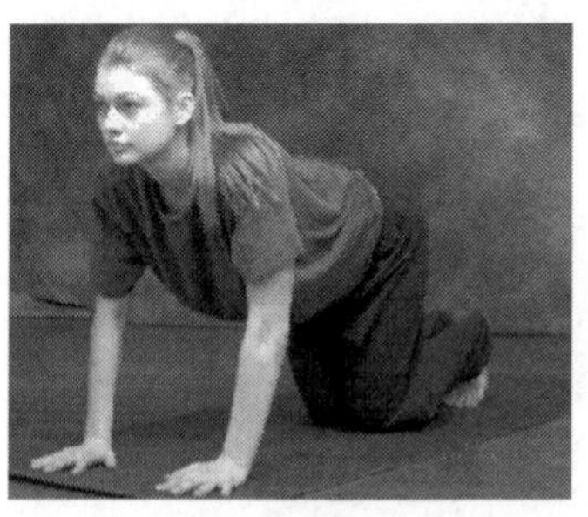

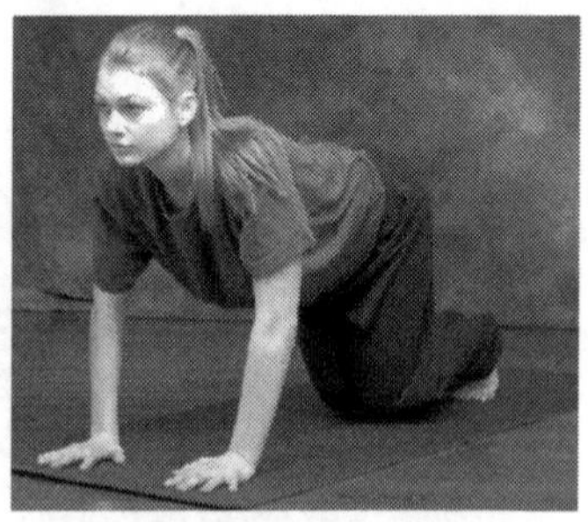

This exercise also works to stabilize the trunk. Engage your core and move the spine as little as possible when lifting the knees up.

- Start on your hands and knees.
- Soften your upper spine gently between the shoulder blades allowing them to soften onto the back.

- Tone the pelvic floor and low belly. Keeping the trunk stable lift your knees one inch off of the floor. Start by holding for three breaths. Try to get up to 10 breaths

7. **Forearm Plank**

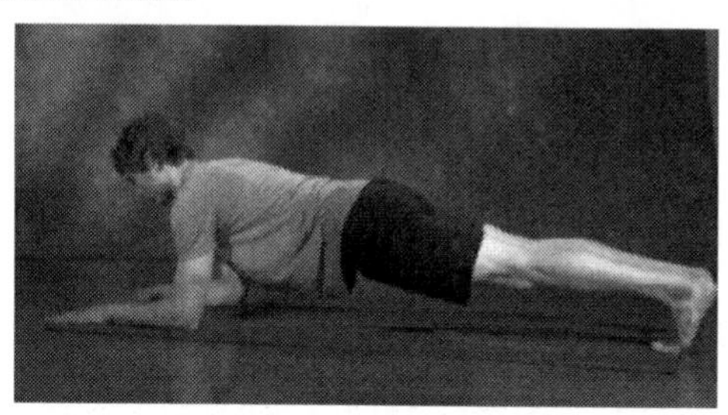

- Lie down on your belly with your elbows under your shoulders and your palms flat to the floor in front of you.
- Lift the hips up off of the floor bringing the ankles, hips, shoulders and ears into one straight line.
- If this is difficult begin by lifting the hips with the knees still on the floor and then try to lift the pelvis up.
- Be aware of the upper back. We have a tendency to round or push up the upper back and use the tightness of our chest muscles to hold us up. Try to broaden the upper chest and let the upper spine soften gently towards the floor.

8. Side Forearm Plank

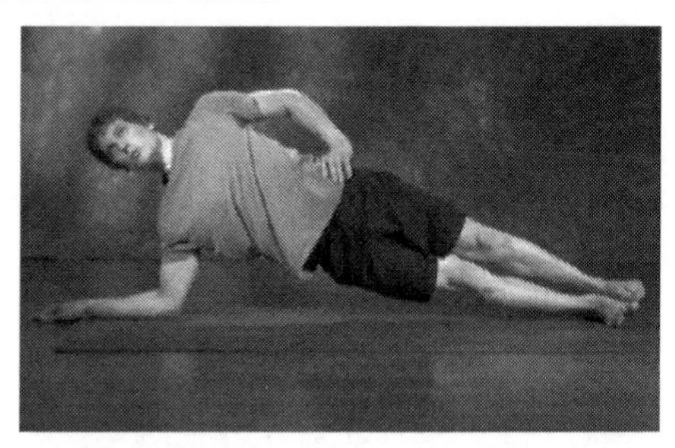

- Lie on your right side with your elbow under your shoulder and your hand lying at a right angle to your trunk with the palm flat to the floor.
- Bring your left hand to your left hip and flex your feet strongly.
- Lift your hips up off the floor trying to create a straight line from your right ankle to hip to shoulder. Do your best to keep your hips stacked on top of one another. The top hip tends to fall backwards.
- If this seems too hard, you can bring your left hand to the floor to try and help with the initial lift.

9. Leg raises on a block

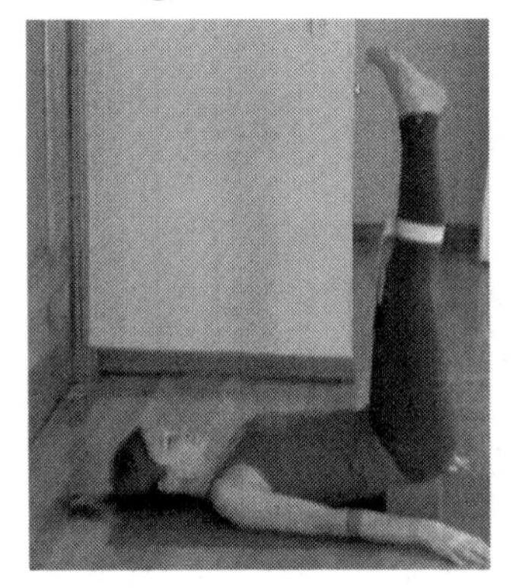

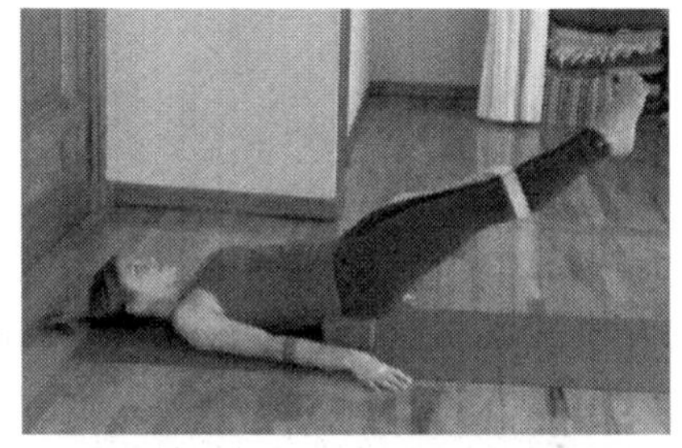

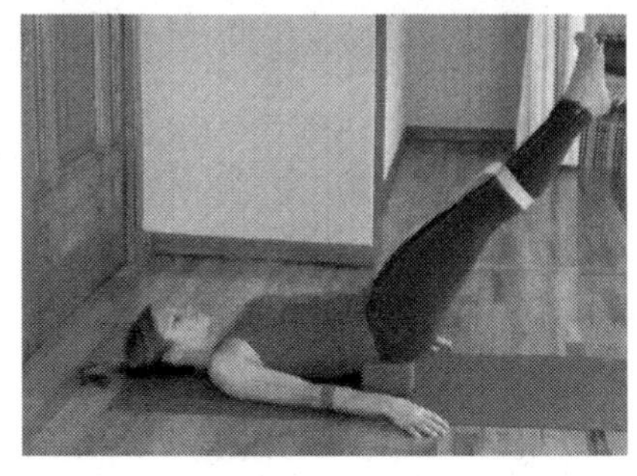

- Lying on your back place a block under your sacrum and tighten a belt around your calves.
- Tone your lower belly and set your lower back in a neutral arch. Try not to shift out of this position
- Lift your legs as high and straight as they will go.
- Trying to keep your trunk solid and steady might be enough work on its own. If it is easy, lower your legs six inches at a time as long as you can keep the spine from shifting its position.

10. Bicycling the Legs

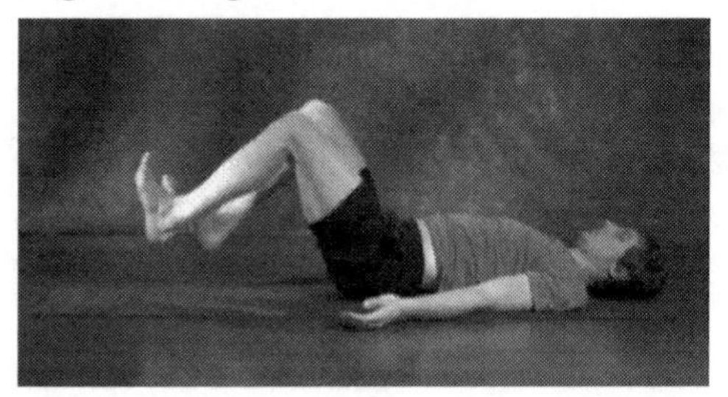

- Lay on your back and draw your right knee into your chest.
- Bring the left foot about a foot off of the floor.
- Begin to switch the position of the legs bring the left knee in and extending the right leg out.
- Try to keep the legs in line with the hips keeping them from extending out to the side.
- Be aware of your inner thighs and try to use them to help initiate the extension of the leg.
- For a tougher exercise, focus on moving the legs at the exact same time so that they cross in the exact middle. The dominant leg wants to move much faster.

11. Six Pack on a Block (Rectus Abdominus)

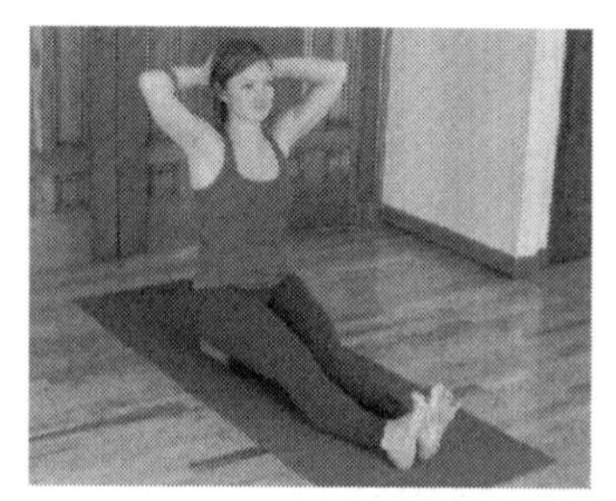
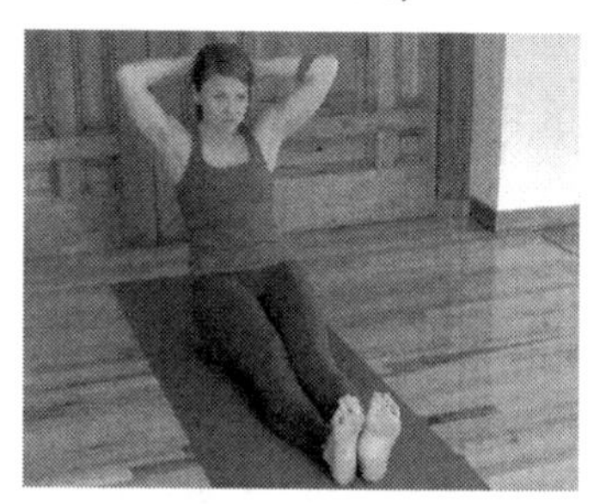

- Sit on a block with your legs outstretched and your fingers interlaced behind your head.
- Begin to lean backwards, shortening the distance between the rib cage and the pelvis engaging the muscle that runs up and down between them. The spine will round slightly into a crunch.
- Keep your heels on the floor. You can bend your knees slightly if the backs of your legs feel tight.
- Once this begins to get easier try to open the elbows wider while keeping the belly muscle engaged. This should bring your back muscles (lats) into play.

12. Switching the Legs

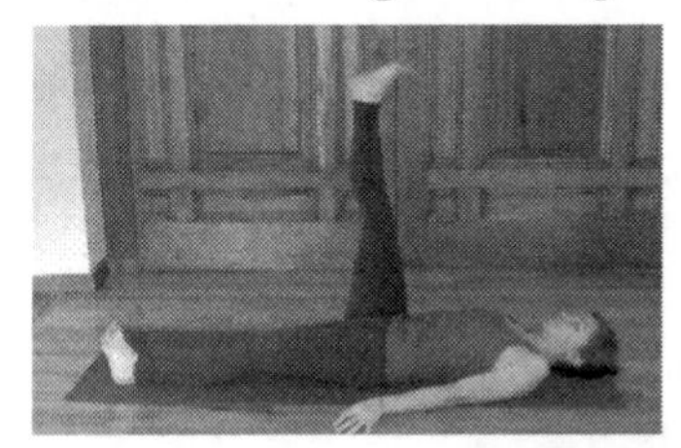

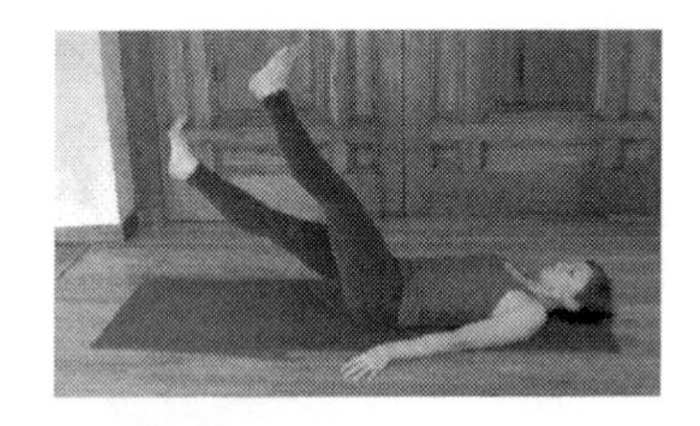

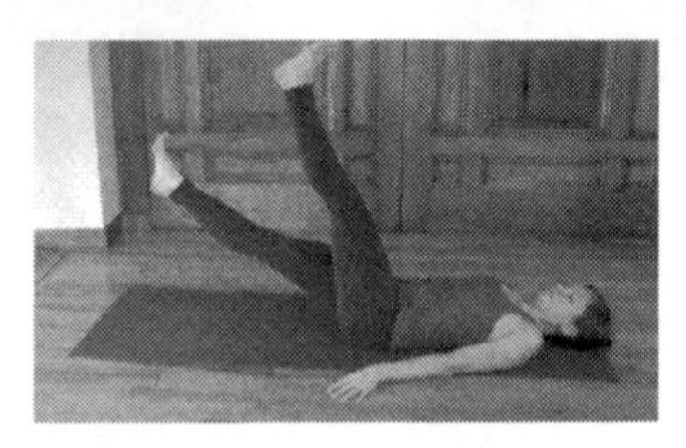

- This is an advanced version of the previous exercise. Try to have as little movement through the trunk as possible.
- Laying flat on your back, tone the core and lift the right leg up to 90°. Activate both legs equally.
- Switch legs at the same time. Try and keep the legs equally straight and balanced side to side. The knees and the toes should always be pointing straight up.
- As this gets easier, try to move the legs at the exact same time crossing at 45°. Your dominant leg is going to want to work way faster than your weaker side.

13. Wall Plank

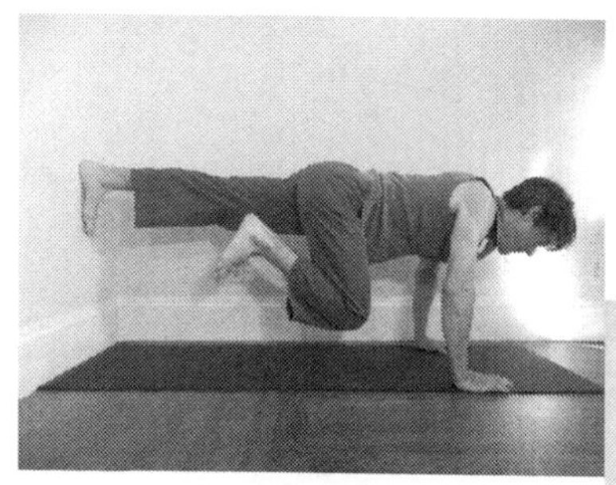

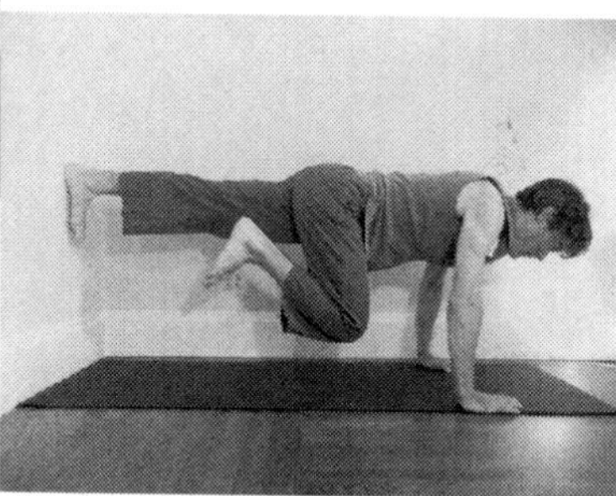

- This is not easy.
- Lay on your belly with your feet up against the base of a wall. Bring your hands up alongside your chest.
- Straighten your arms, and walk your feet up the wall until they're level with your shoulders.
- If you are able to maintain this position, take the right foot off the wall and draw your right knee toward your chest. Maintain a stable trunk.
- Repeat with the left knee.

III The Foot

1. Tennis Ball under foot

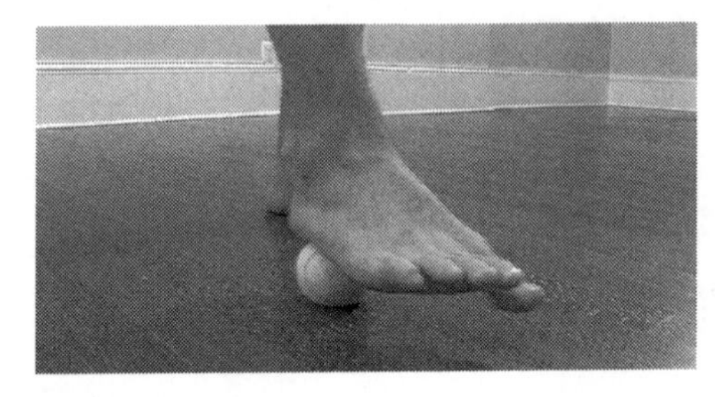

This is a gift to the body that should be with you for years to come. This is great anytime during the day. I recommend keeping a tennis ball in a shoe box under your desk; that will keep the ball from squirting away while you roll.

- Place a tennis ball under your right foot.
- Spend a minute or two rolling the ball under the foot. You can be gentle, or you can apply more pressure. The choice is yours.
- Step off of the tennis ball and bend over your legs. You can check in with your body and see if you feel that the right leg seems a bit longer and looser. Feel free to scan the whole body in this fashion. There is a thick pad of connective tissue on the sole of the foot called the plantar fascia. By releasing the fascia on the underside of the right foot, you effectively release the entire right side of the body.

2. Ankles and Toes

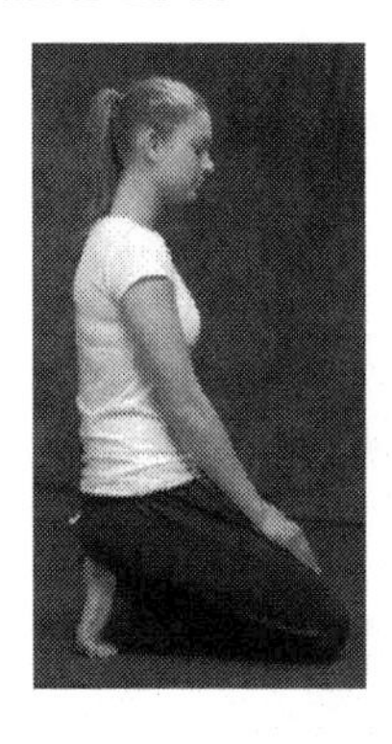

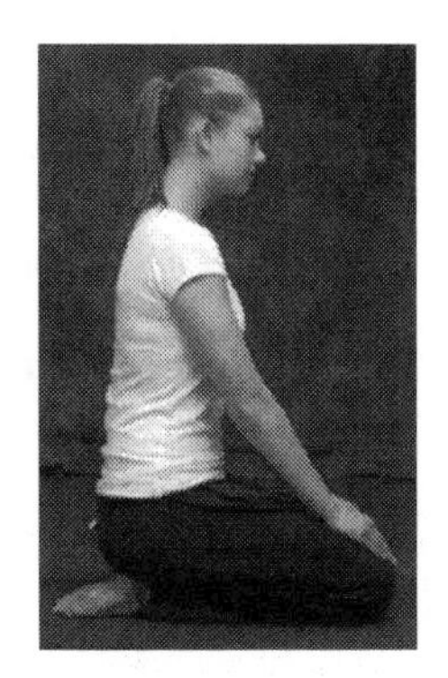

- 1st stage:
  Point your feet bringing the heels as close together as possible. You can even belt the ankles together if you want. Sit on your heels.
- 2nd stage:
  Tuck your toes as far underneath as you can and sit on your heels. Try to have the ball of the foot on the floor and the toes tucked all the way under.

Note: If this is hard in the beginning, put a blanket under your shins and another blanket between your calves and your thighs. It is fine to ease into things over time.

3. Toega

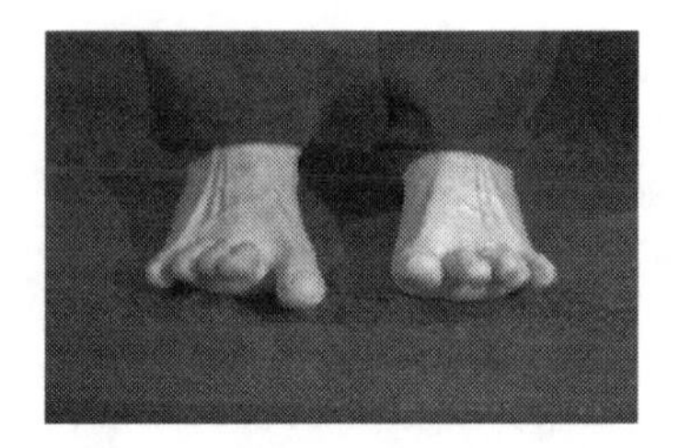

- Lift all ten toes. Spread them apart and try to place them back down with no toes touching.

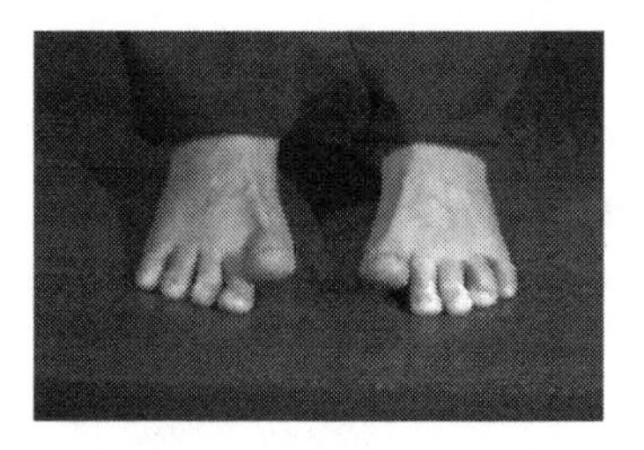

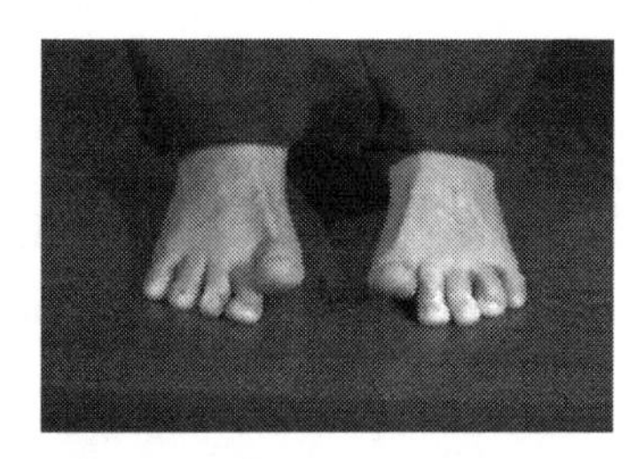

- Lift just the big toes. Place them down. Try lifting them straight up rather than towards the second toe. Even try to draw them closer to each other.

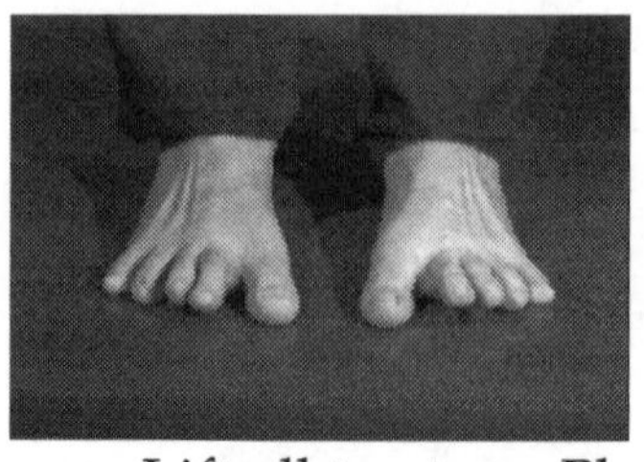

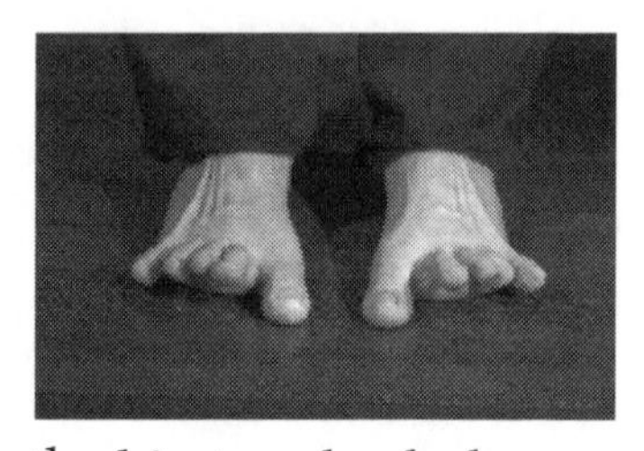

- Lift all ten toes. Place the big toes back down keeping the eight other toes up. Try to place the pinky toe down, keeping the other six toes lifted. Try placing just the fourth toes down next and so on.

- Try lifting the pinky toes by themselves (That's me doing the best I can).

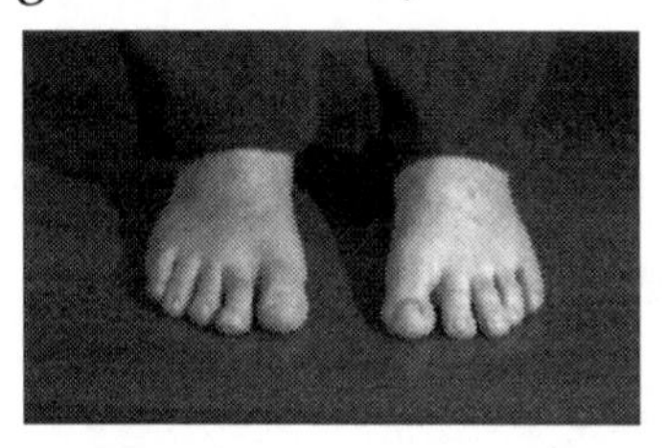

4. Clean House

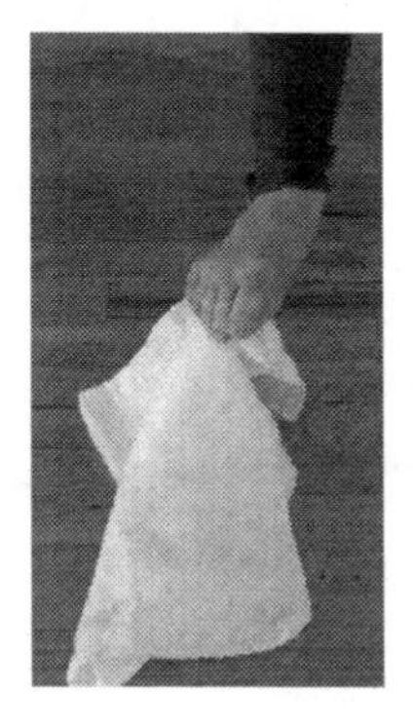

Walk around your house in bare feet and pick objects up off the floor.

5. Heels Up

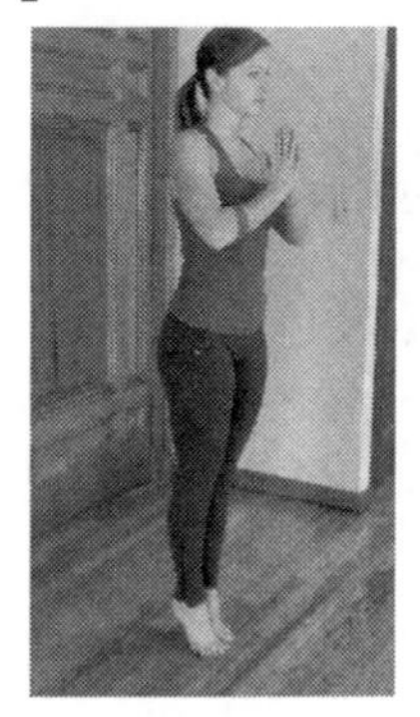

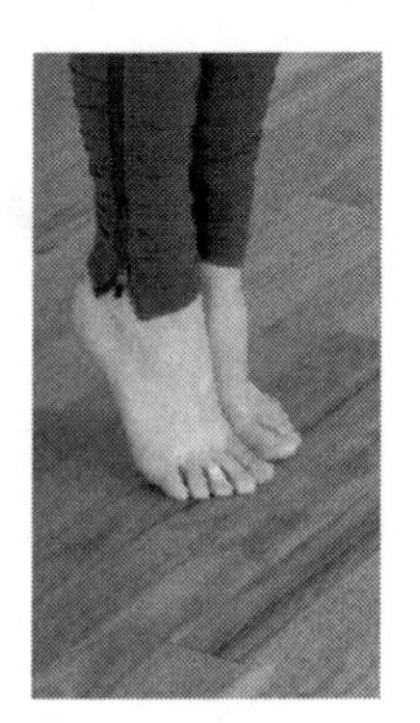

- Stand in bare feet. Keep your big toes together and the heels slightly apart.
- Lift your heels up off the floor balancing on the balls of your feet. Keep the weight to the inside of the foot doing your best to activate the peroneals, the muscles at the outside of the calf.
- Before you come down try to lift a little bit higher and then lower your heels.

IV. The Lower Limb and Pelvis

1. Block between the Thighs at the Wall

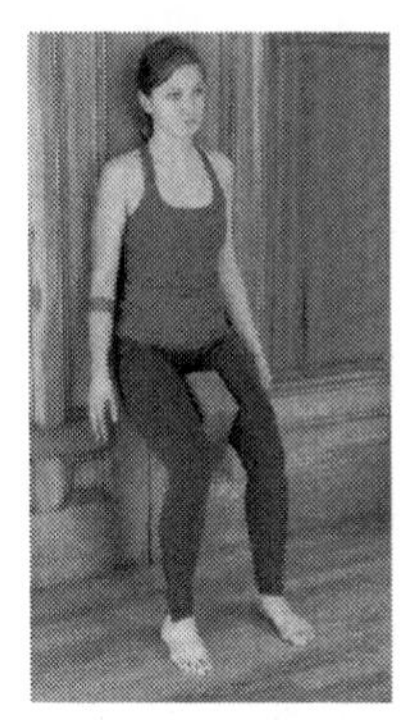
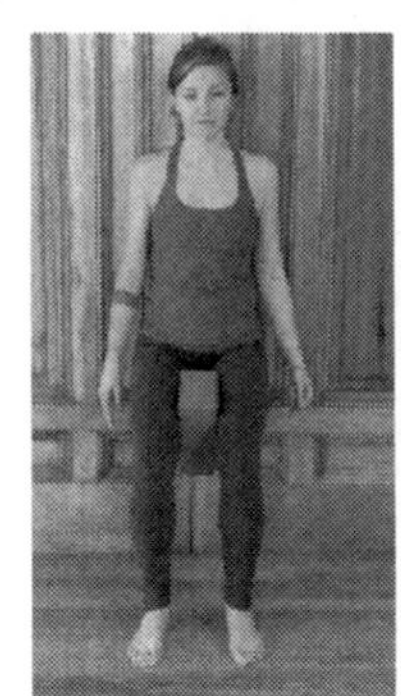

- Stand against a wall placing a block between your inner thighs with your feet 8 or so inches away from the wall.
- Bend the knees and make sure the kneecaps line up with your ankles and your thighs are parallel to each other.
- Engage the inner thigh muscles against the block. Use the top and outside of the thigh at little as possible.

2. Calf Stretch

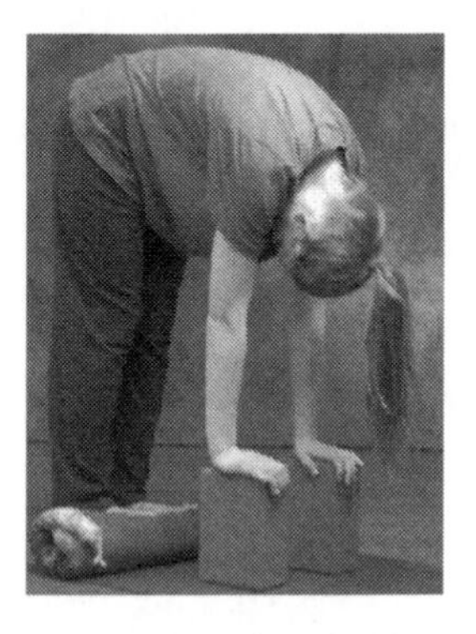

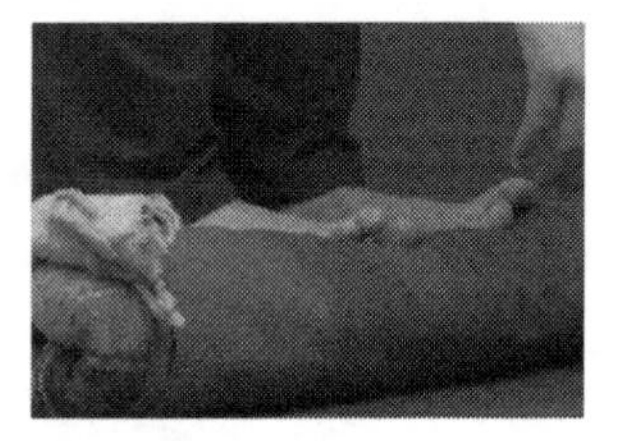

- Roll up a mat or blanket.
- Stand with your feet parallel, your heels on the floor and the balls of your feet as high up the roll as possible.
- Bend your knees softly and lift all ten toes. Keeping your knees aligned over your ankles, bow forward. Have support for your hands if necessary. (A block, or even a chair).
- Stay in this position for a minute or longer.
- Keeping the knees over the ankles, try to bring weight to the inner foot. Lifting your toes will help keep your arches from collapsing.

3. Inner Thighs on the Side

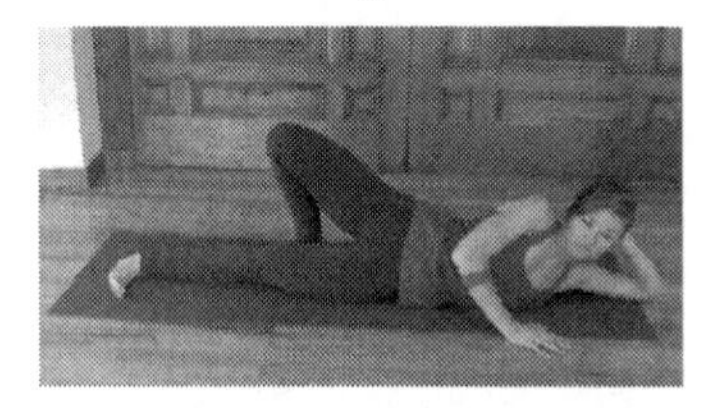

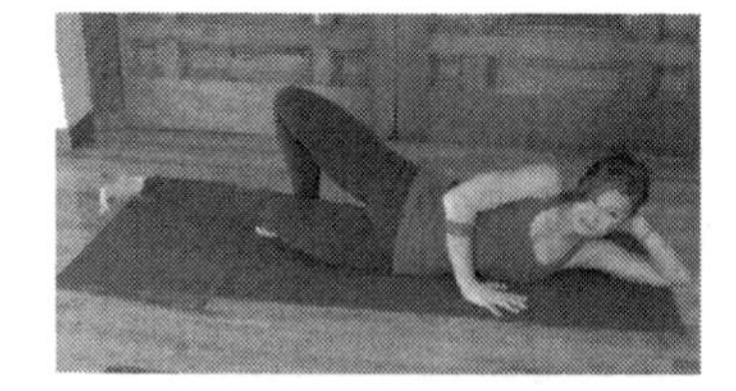

- Lay on your left side with the right knee bent and the right foot flat on the floor in back of the left thigh.
- Lift the extended left leg about 8-10 inches off of the floor.
- Stabilize the pelvis and spine with core muscles and isolate the inner thigh muscle.
- If all of the work seems to be in the thigh and hip bend the knee a little. Make sure to stabilize the pelvis and spine.

4. Binding and Sliding

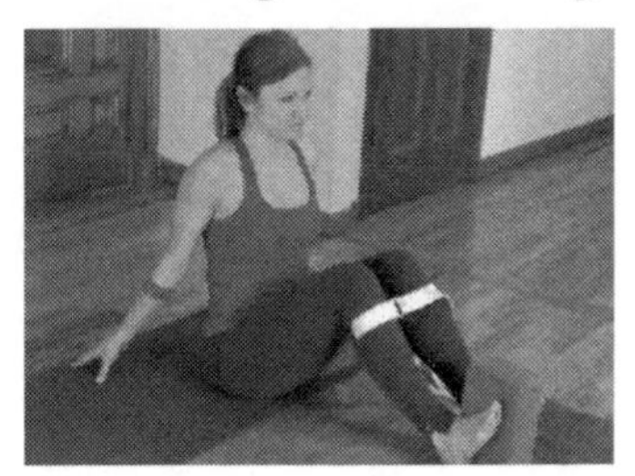

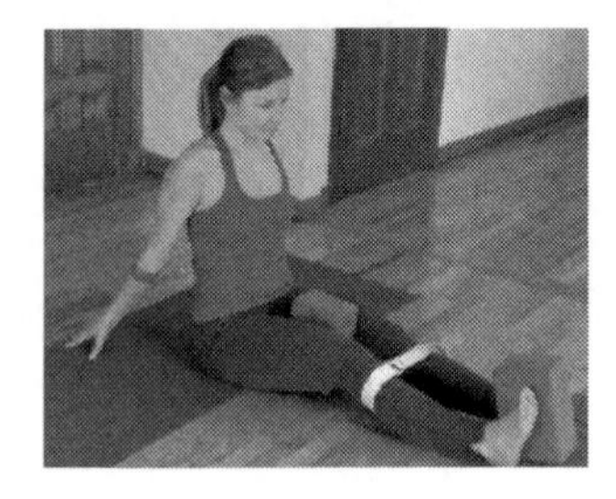

- Place a block between your feet and a block between your inner thighs.
- Keep the big toes on the block and do your best to pull your heels slightly away from the block.
- Belt the calves as tight as you can, a couple of inches below the knee around the meat of the calf muscle.
- Draw the knees towards your chest keeping your heels on the floor. Extend the legs back out.
- Try to keep your feet even, pressing through the inner foot and drawing the outer foot back.
- The emphasis of the exercise is on the inner thigh, outer calf, and mound of the big toe on the inner foot.

5. Glute Stretch on the Back

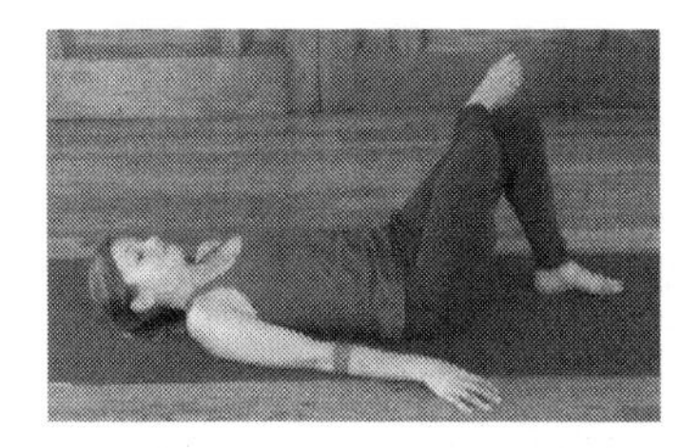

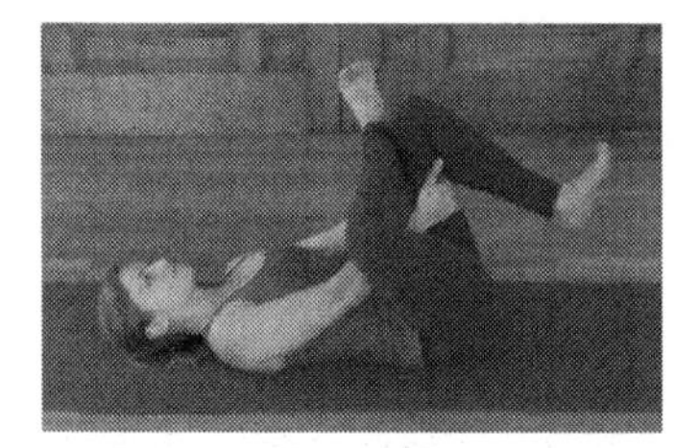

- Lay on your back with the knees bent and your feet flat to the floor.
- Cross the right ankle over the left knee. Flex your right foot. Pick the left foot off of the floor drawing the knee towards you.
- Interlace your fingers behind the left thigh.
- Work to open the right hip energetically moving the hip away from you as the left knee moves closer. Don't push the leg open with your hand.
- Keep your core strong and your lower back in a gentle arch.

6. Piriformis Stretch on the Back

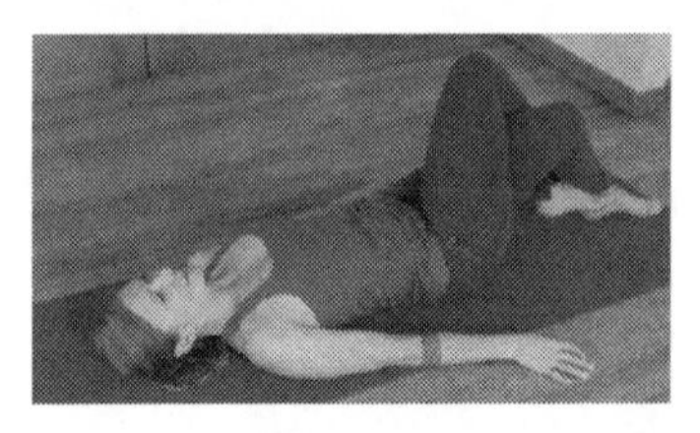
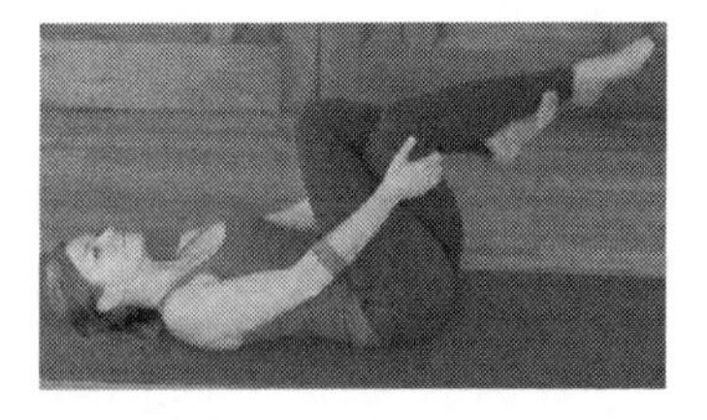

- Lay on your back with the knees bent and your feet flat to the floor.
- Cross the right knee over the left knee. Pick the left foot off of the floor drawing the knee towards you.
- Interlace your fingers in front of the left shin.
- Lengthen the spine, toning your core, trying to bring a gentle curve to the lower back.

7. Low lunge

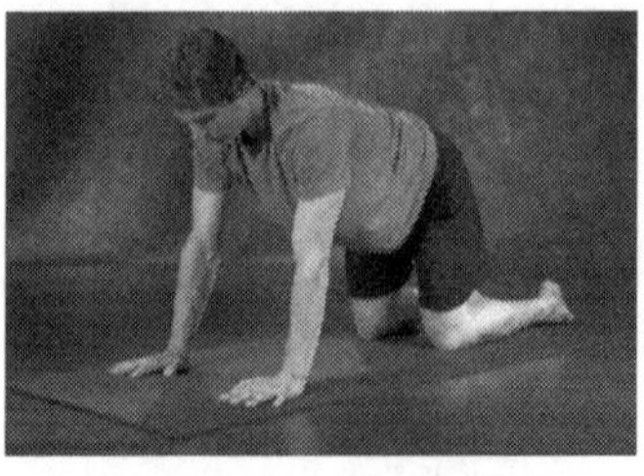
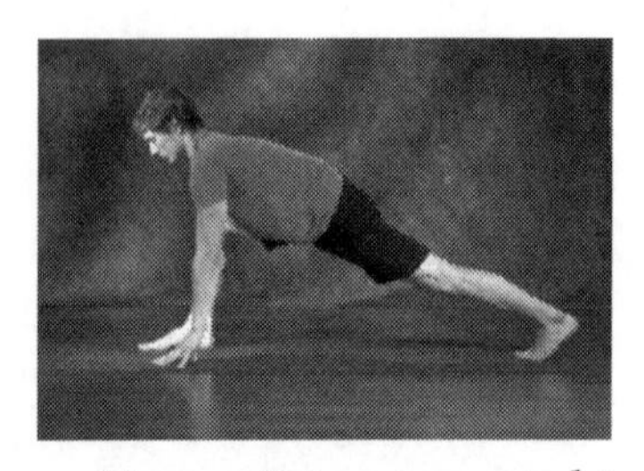

- Starting on your hands and knees bring your right foot forward and straighten your left leg.
- Keep the front knee over the ankle, not past it, and keep your front hip at the height of the knee, not lower.
- Lengthen the spine softening the shoulder blades gently towards each other.

8. Standing psoas stretch

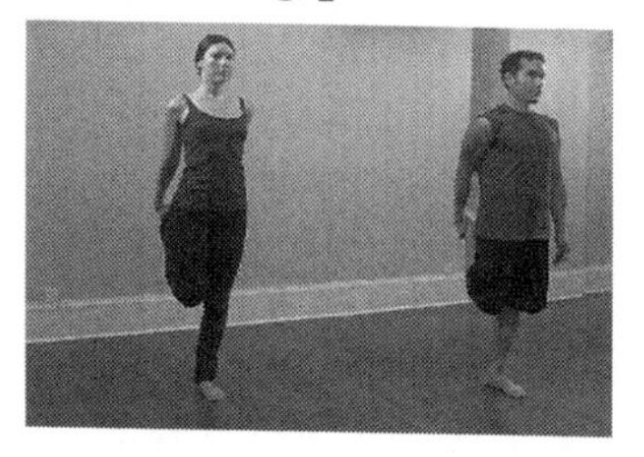

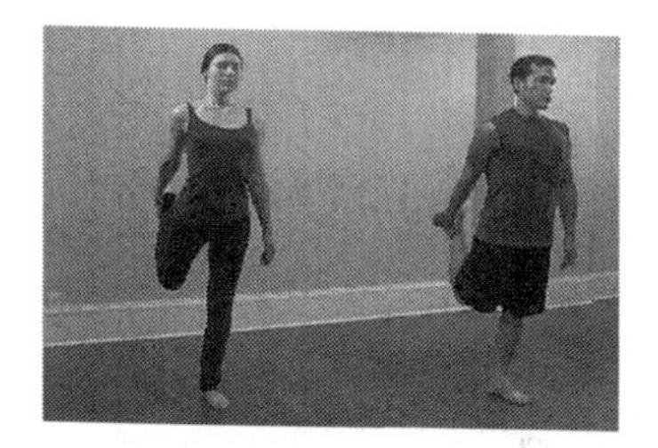

This is a classic standing stretch that also happens to be a deep stretch of the psoas—if it is done correctly. Feel free to use the wall to support yourself.

- Bend your right leg behind you and take hold of the right foot or ankle with your right hand. Bring your knees in line with one another, keeping the heel in line with your sit bone. If your outer hip is very tight it won't be easy to keep the knees in line.
- Pull the right leg behind you gently. Keep the pelvis and shoulders facing forward and upright the whole time.
- Keep the pelvic floor and the low belly strong as you try to pull the leg behind you through the balanced action of the inner and outer thigh.

If you have tight hips, it will be difficult to keep the legs aligned as you draw the right leg back. The knee will pull sideways, and it is imperative that you keep the legs in line. This is an issue with the iliotibial tract, or IT band, not the psoas, but as we know, everything is connected (no pun intended).

9. Extended side angle

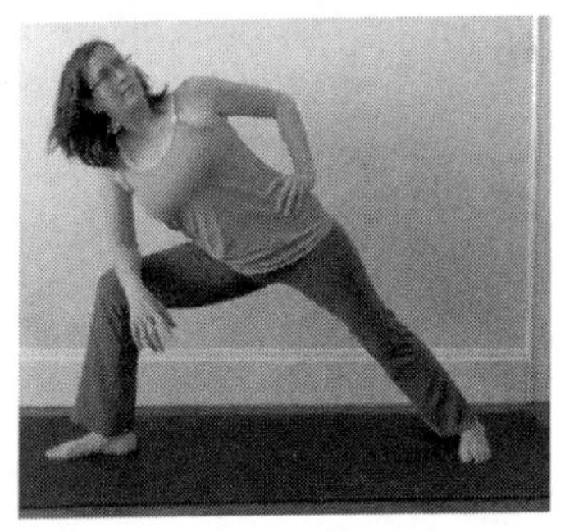

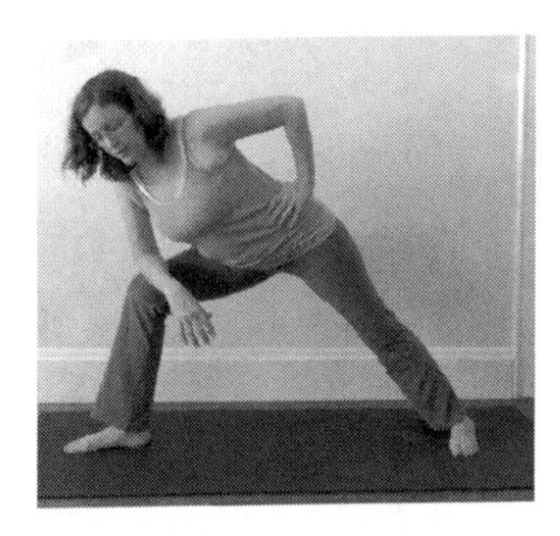

- Stand with the feet as far apart as is comfortable.
- Point the right foot and turn the left foot in a little.
- Bend the right knee, bringing the right forearm onto the right thigh and the left hand onto the left hip.
- Rotate your pelvis back, allowing the left inner thigh to move back, lining up the outer left hip with the left ankle bone. This should pitch your upper body forward a little and create a deep crease in your hips.
- Keeping the legs stable, try to bring the trunk on top of the legs without tucking the pelvis back under. This will require a lot of tone in the pelvic floor and lower abdomen. Don't allow the left thigh to move forward.

10. Runners Stretch

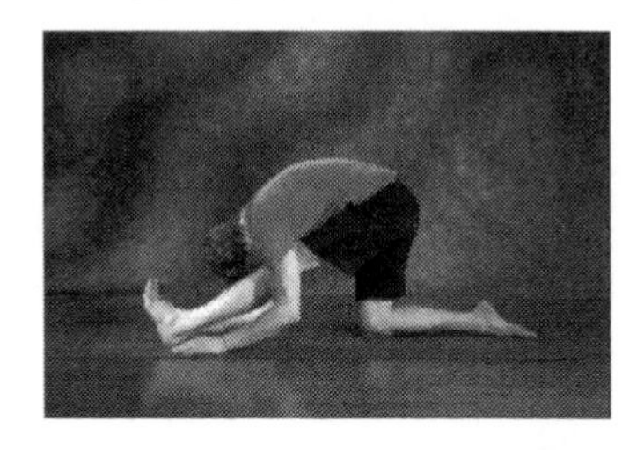

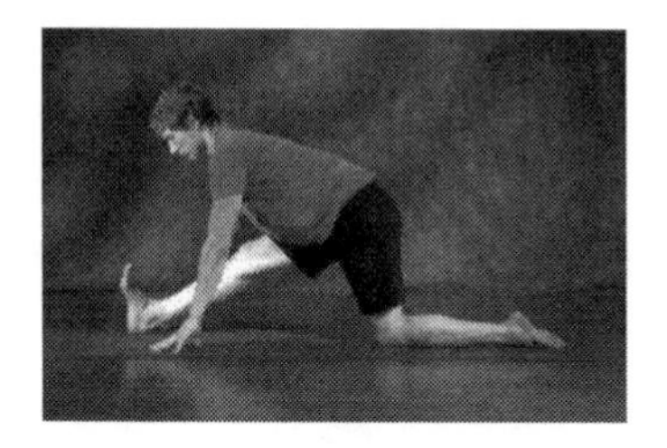

This is one of the deeper hamstring stretches.

- Start on your hands and knees
- Step your right foot forward far enough to extend it straight with the foot flexed off of the floor and the pelvis on top of the left knee.
- This is a deep stretch of the hamstring so use blocks for the hands if that helps you to find a flat back.
- Square the hips and try to extend to the spine forward over the right leg.

11. Dying Warrior

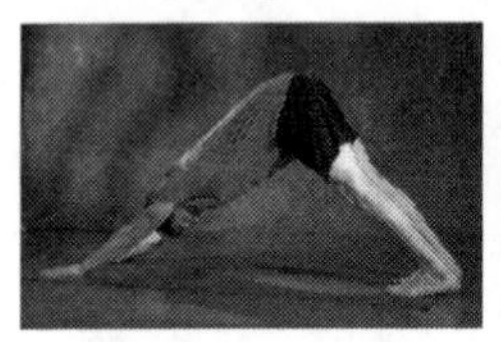
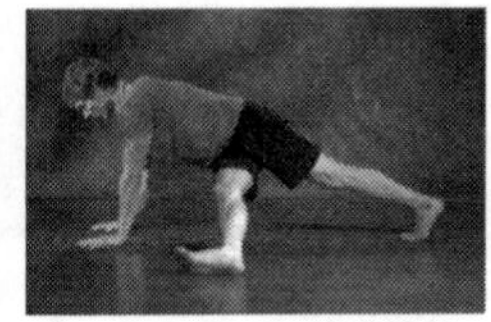
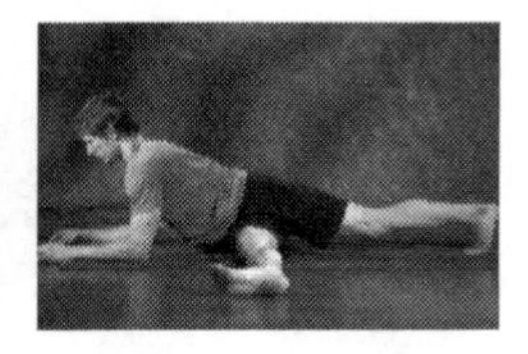

- Starting on your hands and knees or in downward facing dog, bring the right leg across the leg side of the body, trying to swing it slowly up to the height of the pelvis or higher.
- Stay in the position of the second picture for a few breaths before you come down to the ground. This is a stretch of the outer hip that we love more than most.
- When one hip is on the ground work on turning the other (top) hip towards the foot on the floor. The stretch will likely move from the outer hip to the area between the pelvis and the rib cage.

12. Sitting On A Chair, Lean Forward With Flat Back

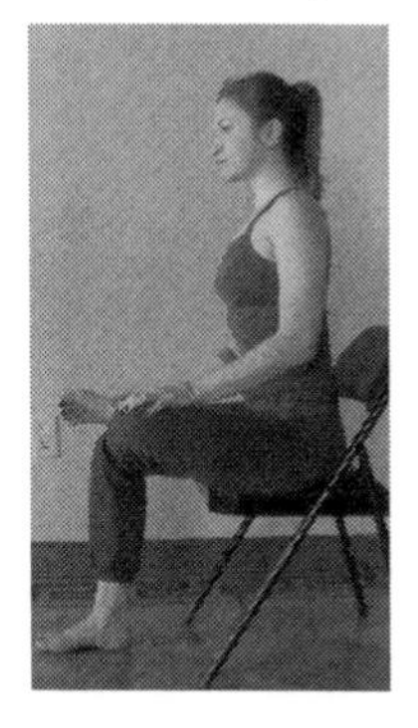
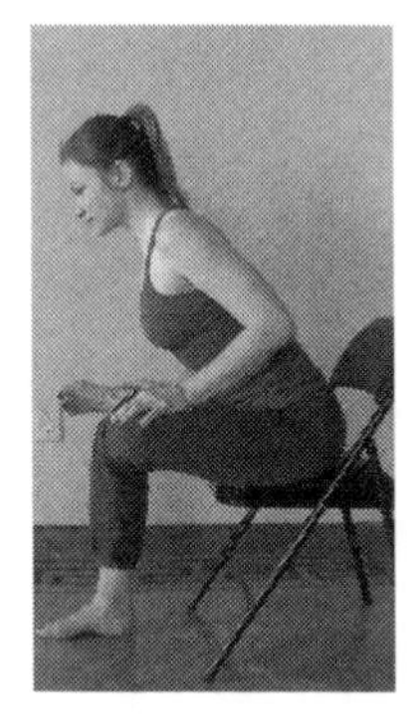

- Sit upright in a chair with a flat back.
- Cross the right ankle over the left knee. Flex the right foot (push through the heel).
- Begin to lean forward keeping the natural arches in the back (meaning don't round forward and collapse your chest).
- If the lower back begins to round backwards, stop. You have gone to far. Go back to a point where you can keep the curve in the lower back and breath here.

13. Ankle To Knee Forward Bend

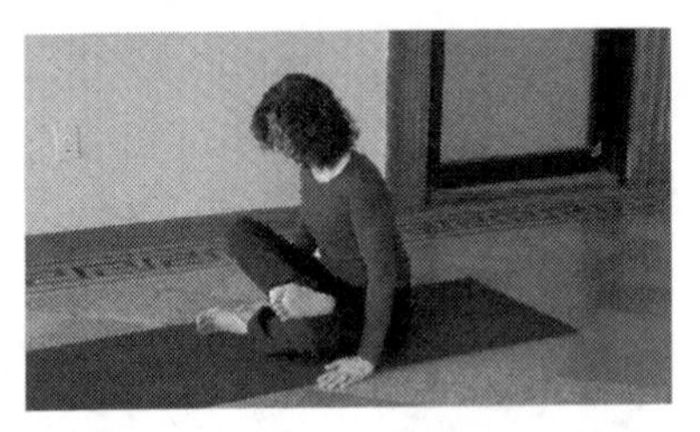

This stretch happens in two parts depending on what you feel in the first part.

- Sit with the legs straight out in front of you. Cross the right ankle over the left knee. Try to not to excessively round the back. Feel the natural curves in the spine. Lift the chest and lean forward. If you feel this in your piriformis (side of the butt) this is as far as you'll go. Take deep breaths and then change sides. If you feel this in your hamstring (back of the leg) move onto the second stage.
- Keep your right ankle on top of your left knee and bend the left knee placing the left ankle below the right knee. (It's a deeper version than sitting "cross-legged".)
- Try and stack your shins on top of one another, right shin on top. The left shin should be hiding underneath the right shin.

- Stay even on both sit bones. Most people need to press their hands down, lift the butt up, and then place the butt down again taking the sit bone off the leg that's on top down to the floor first.
- Flex the feet strongly and try to avoid letting the top ankle collapse down into the leg that's below it.
- If you look down between your legs there should be a triangle of open space, the legs should be right on top of one another.

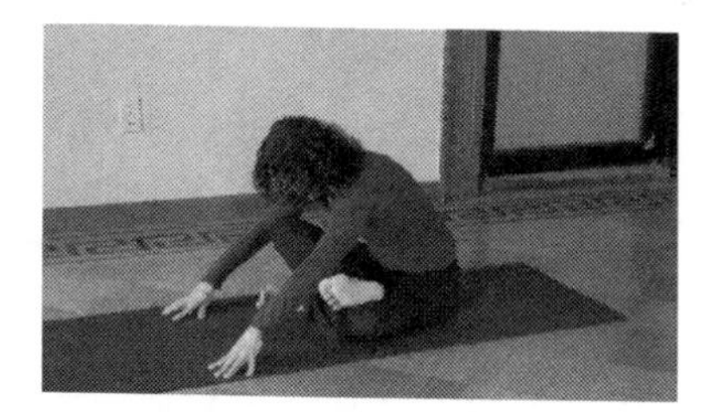

- Extend forward stretching deep into the piriformis. Breath.
- Do the other side.

14. Standing Pigeon

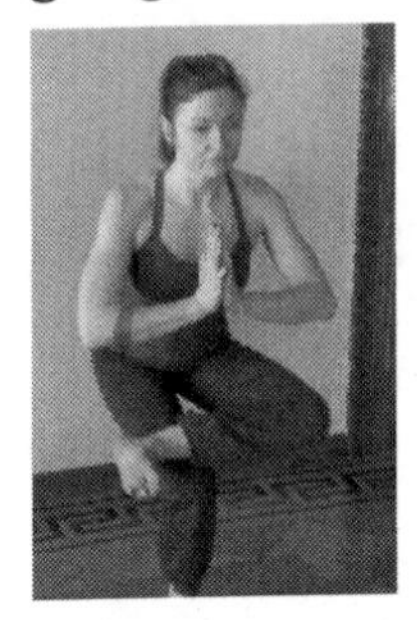
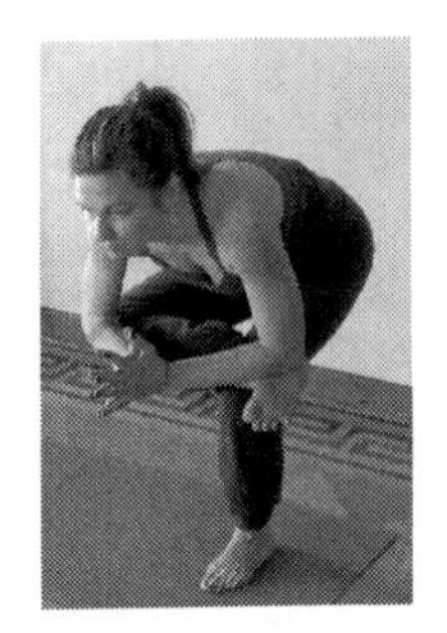

- Stand with the feet hip distance apart and parallel.
- Cross the right ankle over the left knee. Flex the right foot strongly (push through the heel).
- Begin to squat. Think about lowering down backwards more than leaning forward. Stick the butt out.
- If you can bring the forearms onto the right shin, place them there and hold.
- Ideally the right shin is parallel to both the front of your mat and the floor.
- Breath.
- Change sides.

15. Pigeon

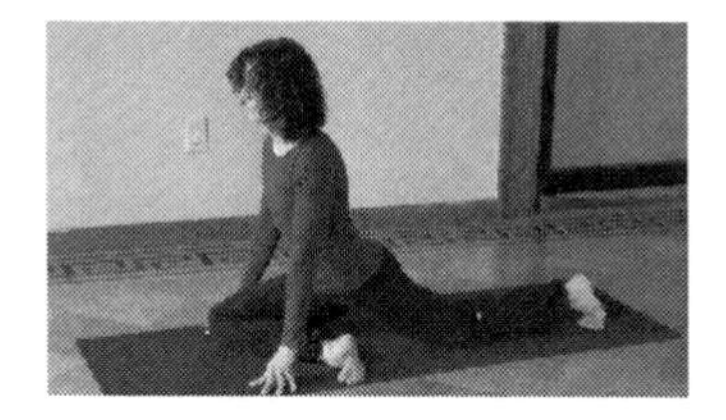

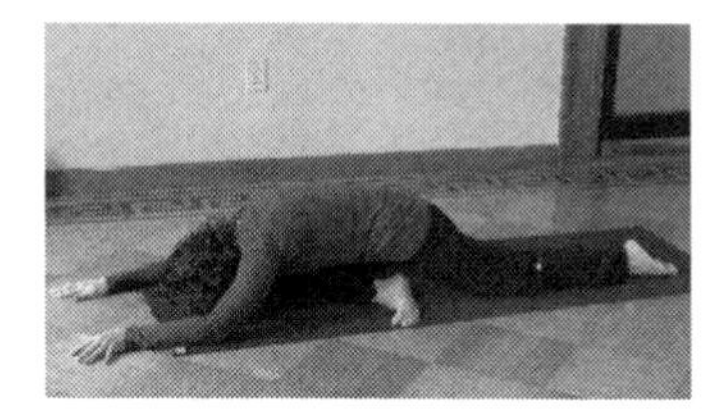

- Starting on your hands and knees slide your right knee towards your right wrist. Make sure that your right foot moves forward enough to get to the outside of the left thigh. If you fall onto the outside of your right hip, you may need to support that hip with a pillow or folded blanket.
- Slide the left leg straight back and make sure that the ankle is lined up with the knee and hip and that the foot is pointed straight.
- Walk the hands back alongside the hips and then try to and bring your hips towards square. (You will see that when the right leg is in front, the right hip pulls forward. Try to pull the right hip back and bring the left hip forward. You will probably feel more in your right hip as you do this.)
- Bow forward keeping the arms active and find the stretch deep in the right buttock. Take many breaths here.
- Change sides.

16. Butt Stretch

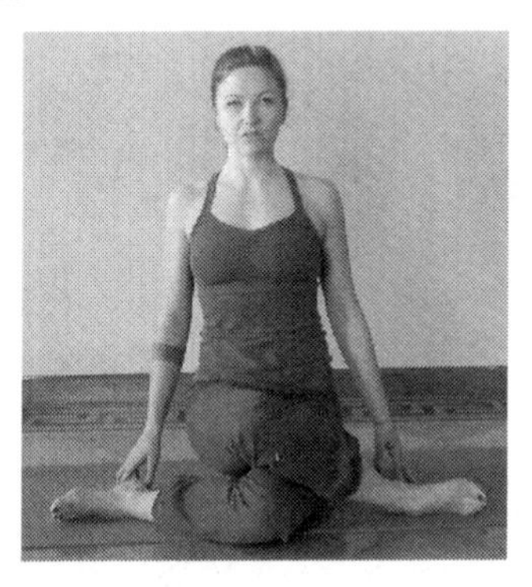

You might want to sit up on a block or a few pillows or folded blankets (or towels) to begin this stretch.

- Come onto your hands and knees. Put your right knee in front of your left, both feet sticking out to the sides of you.
- Sit back between your feet onto your support.
- Try to keep the right knee on top of the left. For many of us it will lift and move to the right a bit. That's fine.
- Bow forward. If this seems relatively doable, lower the support. If that is also easy, sit your butt on the floor.
- Breathe.
- Change sides.

17. Twist on Back

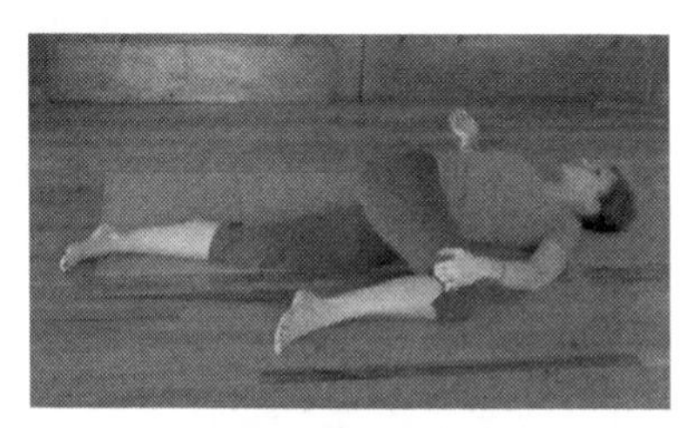

- Lay flat on your back.
- Draw the right knee into the chest and keep the left leg extending long on the floor. The left toes point straight up towards the ceiling.
- Begin to twist drawing the right knee across the left side of the body. The right knee can go over as much as possible, even reaching the floor if that work (or you could put a block or blanket or pillow under it).
- Let the left hand rest on the right thigh. Reach your right arm out to the right.
- Keep tone in the belly and look over the right shoulder. Slow down the breath and let the stretch happen.
- Change sides.

18. Squats

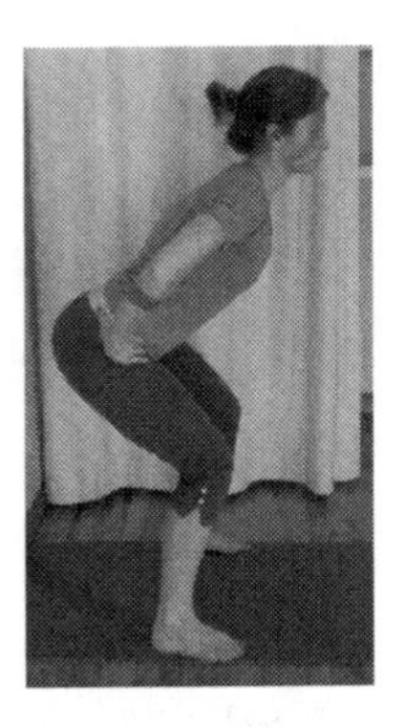

- Stand up straight with feet shoulders-width apart or slightly wider. Keep the feet as close to parallel as possible making sure to work equally on both sides. Feel free to hold onto a chair as you begin to explore this exercise.
- Slowly and steadily bend your knees and flex your hips to lower your butt toward the floor. Don't let your knees move forward of the toes. You are trying to squat down backwards.
- Don't worry about how far down you can go at first. Work on maintained alignment and a pain free descent.
- Lower down to the best of your ability and hold for five breaths. Try to increase this over time to 25 breaths.

- An advanced variation is to isolate and engage your pelvic floor muscles while squatting. In this version you try to tone the levator ani (a thick muscle at the top of the pelvic floor. The pelvic floor consists of three layers, the sphincters, the perineum and the all important levator ani) for both lowering into the squat and lifting back up. This creates both eccentric and concentric contraction of deep muscles. Muscles work in a number of ways. They can engage and contract (concentric), engage and expand (eccentric), and engage without moving (isometric). That can help ease the strain on the piriformis.

V. Shoulders, Chest and Neck

1. Back Stretch on the Belly

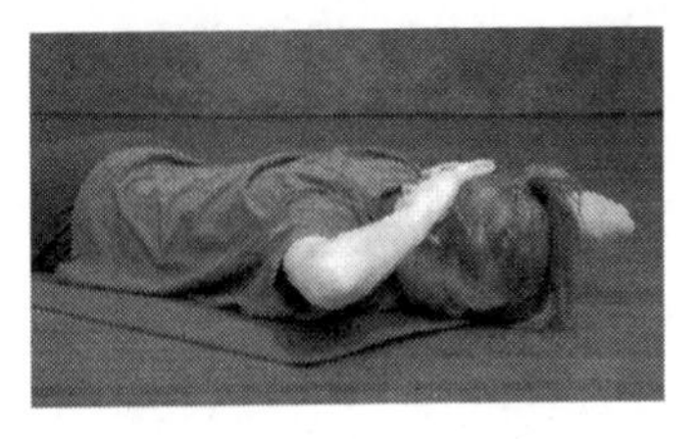
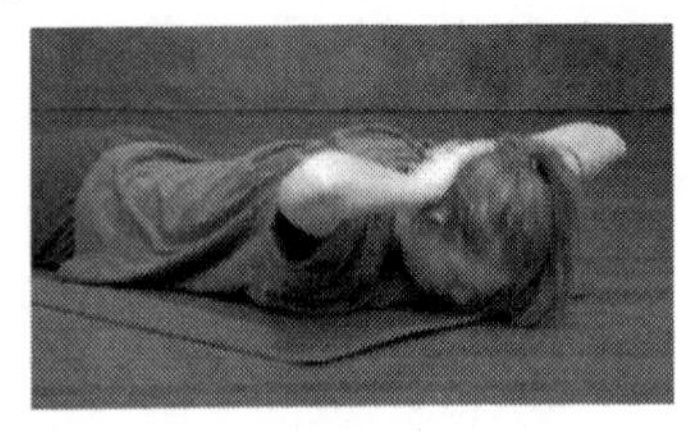

- Lie on your stomach. Interlace your fingers behind your head and lengthen the back of your neck up into your fingers.
- Draw the belly in and lift your trunk up off the floor, keeping your chin soft. The head, neck and chest should move in one piece.
- The elbows want to move up and out as you lift up. Let the hands rest on the head without pushing the head forward.

2. Winged Victory

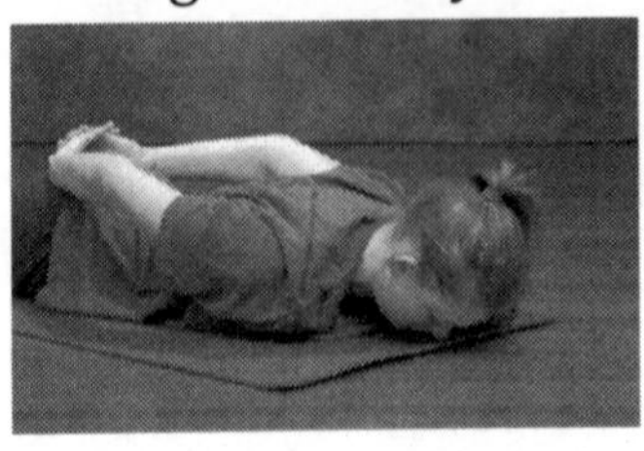
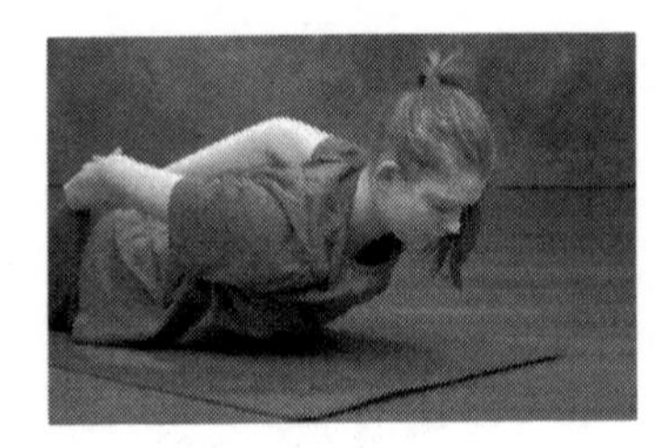

- Lie on your stomach. Interlace your fingers behind your back. Lengthen the back of your neck looking straight down.

- Draw the belly in and lift your trunk up off the floor, keeping your chin soft. You want the head, neck, and chest to move in one piece.

3. Belt Stretch

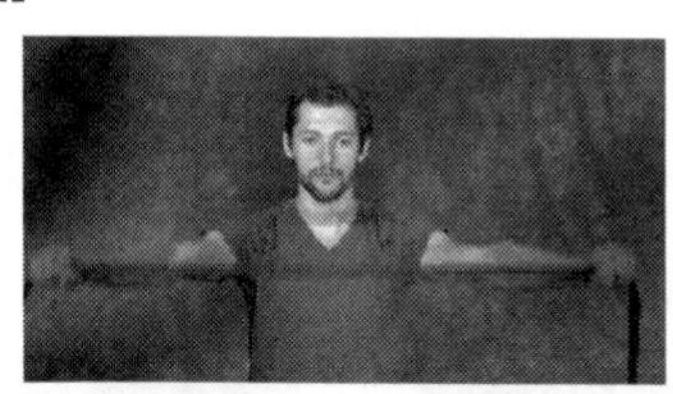

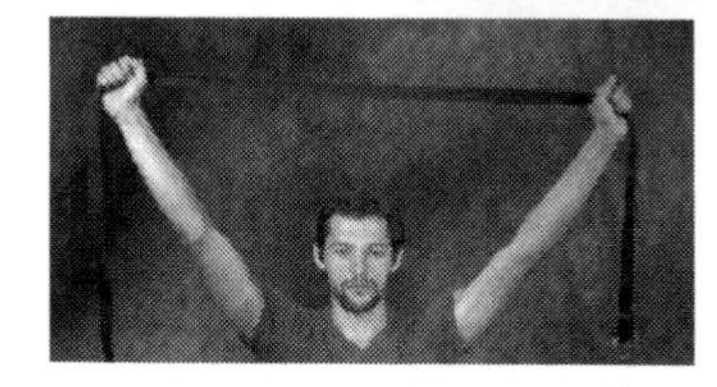

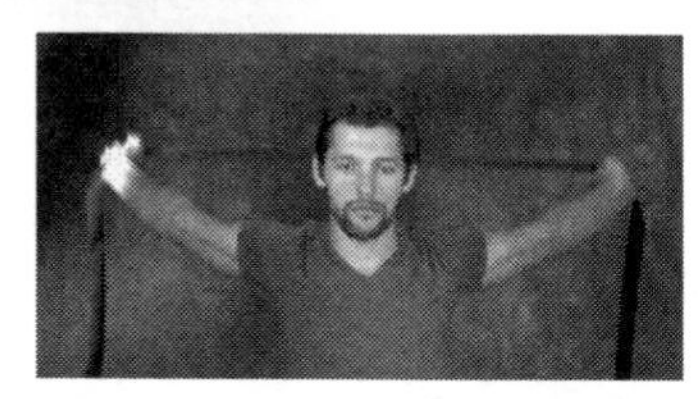

This is a strong stretch of the Pectoralis minor at the front of the chest.

- Hold a belt or a broom stick with your hands wide apart. Bring the belt over your head and behind you keeping the arms straight. You may need to move your hands slightly further apart for them to stay straight.
- The key is for the head, neck and chest to remain still.
- Try to move both arms at the same pace.
- As this gets easier move the hands closer together.

4. Block Over Head

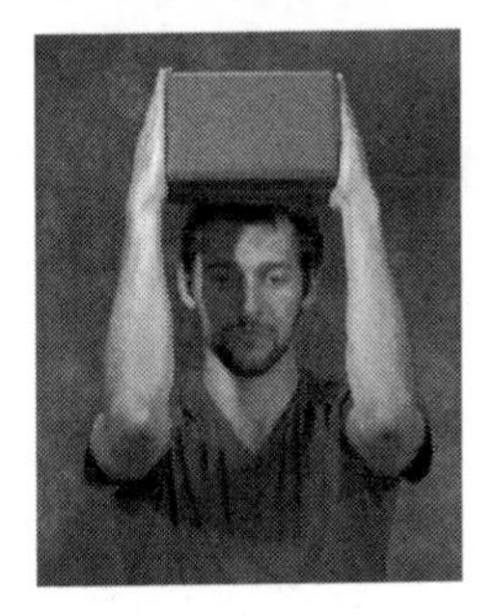
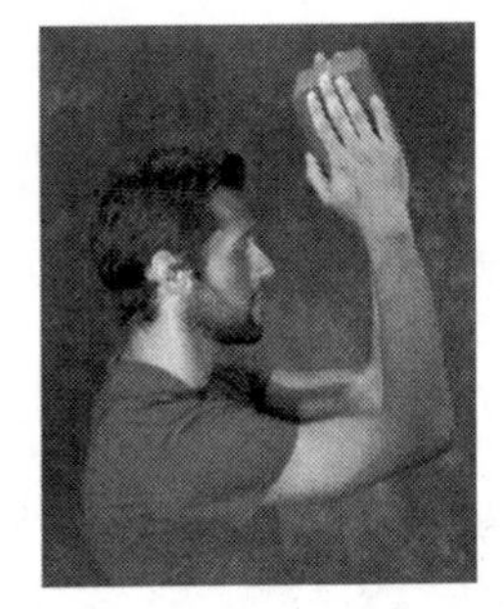
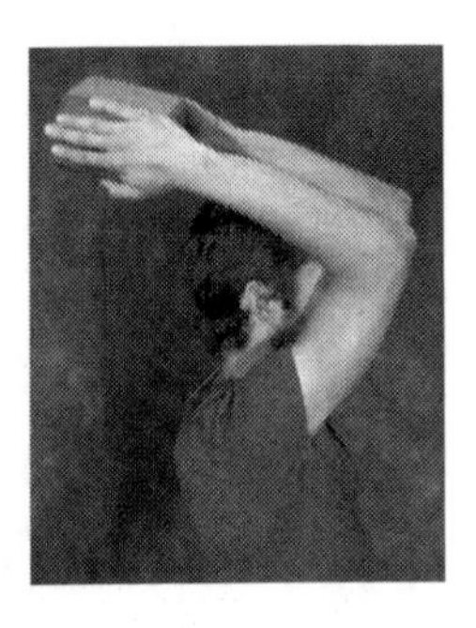

- Hold a block in your hands with your arms bent at 90 degrees.
- Keep your elbows in line with the wrists. You can belt the arms just above the elbow if you'd like.
- Raise your arms and the block up keeping the arms bent at the right angle.
- Engage the abdominals so that your rib cage is stabilized throughout. Don't let your rib cage puff forward.
- Try to keep the elbows parallel, making sure they don't flare out to the side.

5. Eagle Arms

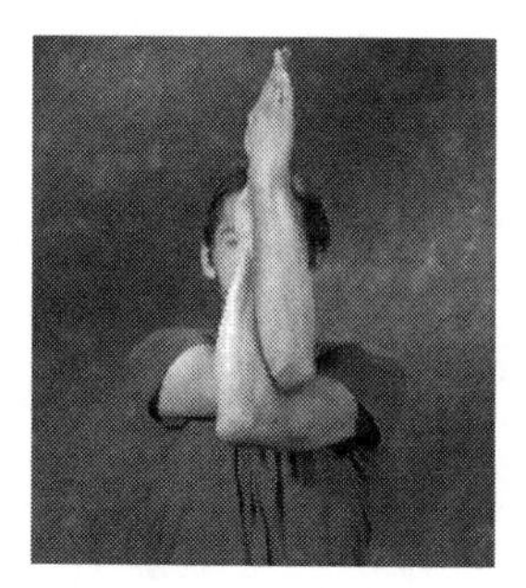

- Bring the right arms underneath the left arm, crossing the elbows.
- Try drawing the forearms close to each other and if possible get the right fingers to press into the left palm.
- Lift the elbows up to the height of the shoulders and keep the forearms in line with your nose.
- Press the hands together to activate the muscles of the shoulders and at the same time try to pull the shoulder blades towards each other on the back.

6. Elbows Apart

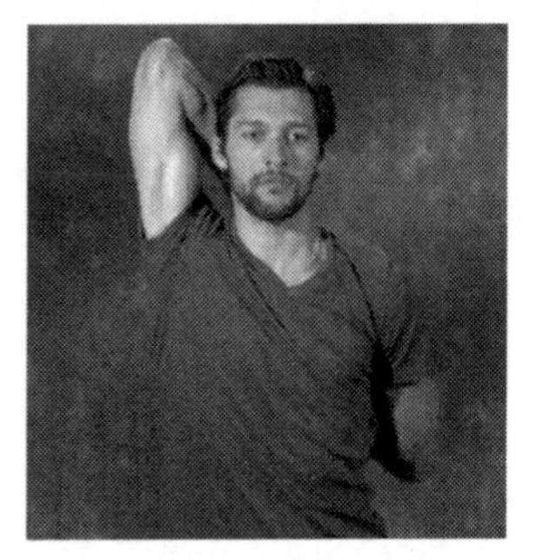

- Lift your right arm up and turn you right hand to face behind you. You can bring your left hand up to assist in the rotation of the upper arm towards the back of the body.
- Bend the elbow and drop your right hand behind your back.
- Bring the left arm out to the side, slightly in front of the chest, and turn the palm towards the back of the body and try to bring the left hand towards your back and maybe even to interlace with the fingers of the right hand. Feel free to use a belt to assist you.
- Muscularly pull everything towards the midline of the body, with the upper arms moving towards parallel and the elbows moving away from each other towards the floor and the ceiling.

7. Pectoralis Major & Minor

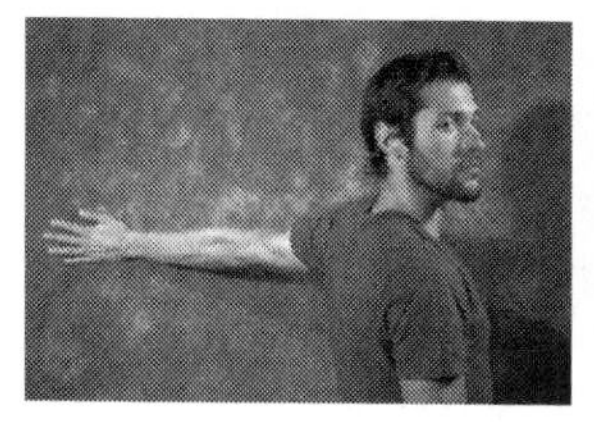
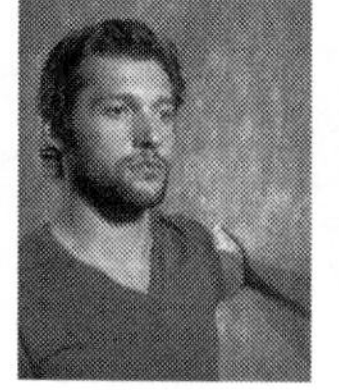
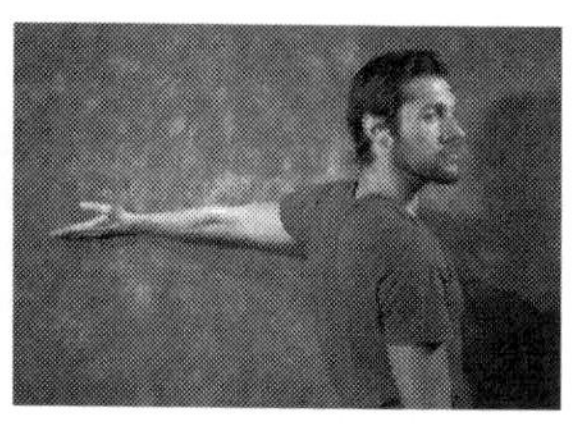

This is a classic stretch that is easy to find variations for (standing in a doorway with your arms on either side of the frame, and stretch forward). The muscle that stretches when the palm is turned up is pectoralis minor, one of the tighter muscles of the upper body.

- Stand 8-12 inches from the wall with the side of your body towards the wall. Extend your arm behind you with the palm against the wall at the height of your shoulder.
- Turn your feet and torso 45 degrees away from the wall.
- Keeping the arm well connected, stretch across the upper chest.
- Return to the beginning, torso facing forward with the side of the body facing the wall. Turn your palm to face up with your pinky finger against the wall at the height of your shoulder and repeat the stretch. This should be a shorter and sharper stretch of pectoralis minor.

8. QL on the Floor

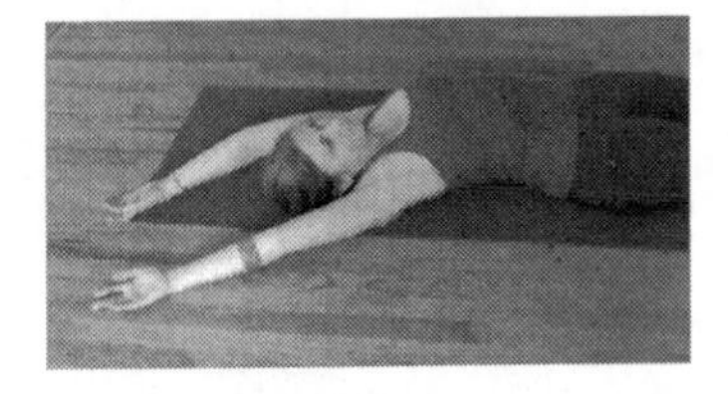

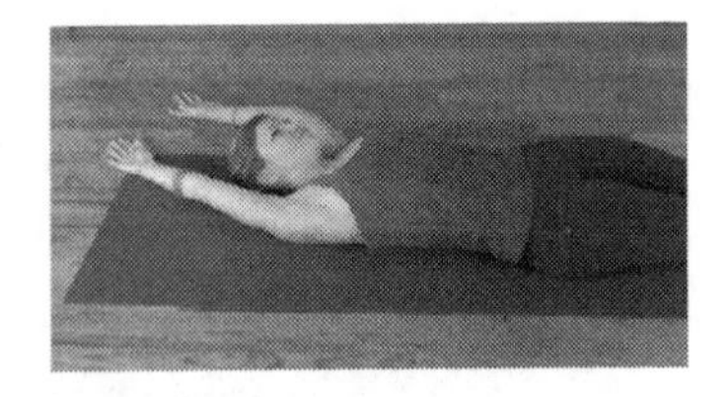

- Laying on your back extend your arms over your head.
- Stabilize your legs and pelvis and arc your trunk to the side
- You want to lengthen and stretch the area between the pelvis and the rib cage.

9. Rotator Cuff Strengthener

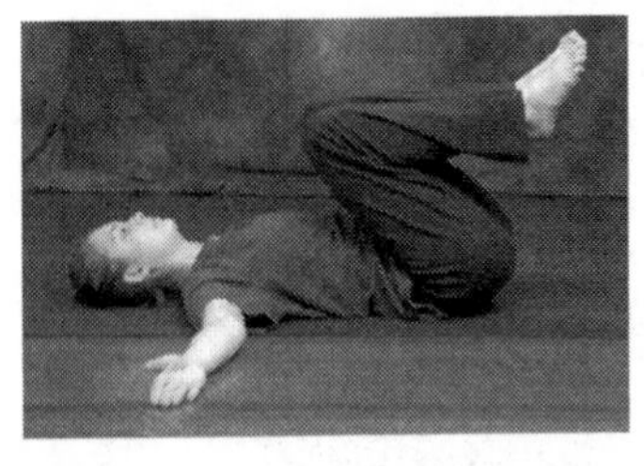

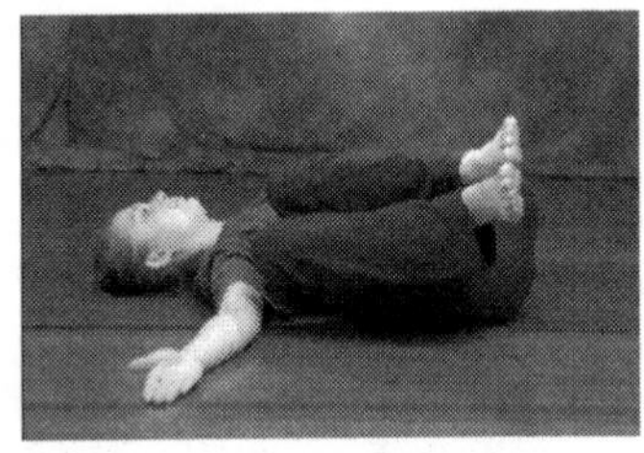

This is the same shape as the earlier core twist only now the focus is on stabilizing the muscles of the rotator cuff onto the back.

- Lie on your back on the floor with your arms outstretched from your shoulders, like the letter T, palms facing the ceiling.
- Bend your knees and bring them towards your chest. Twist, moving your knees towards your

right inner elbow on an angle. Stay grounded in the left shoulder.

- The key to strengthening the rotator cuff is to not letting the shoulders lift off the floor.
- An advanced variation is to work with straight legs.

10. Side Stretch

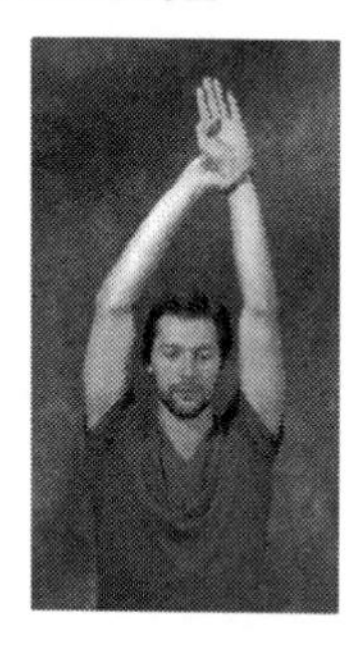
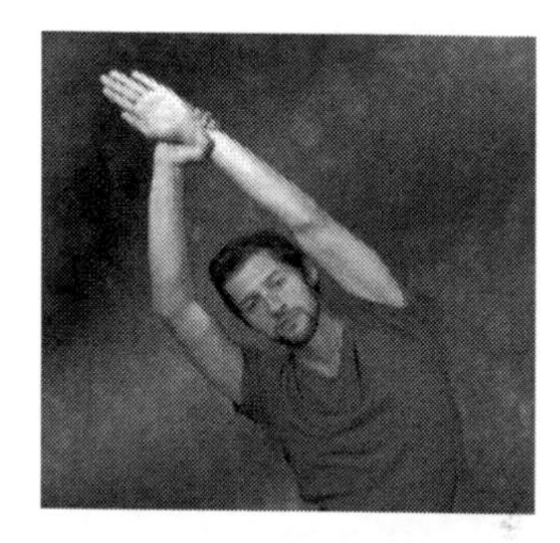

- Bring both hands over head. Stabilize the legs and pelvis. The pelvis should be pointing straight forward. Take hold of the right wrist in the left hand.
- Stretch to the left.

11. Sub Occipital

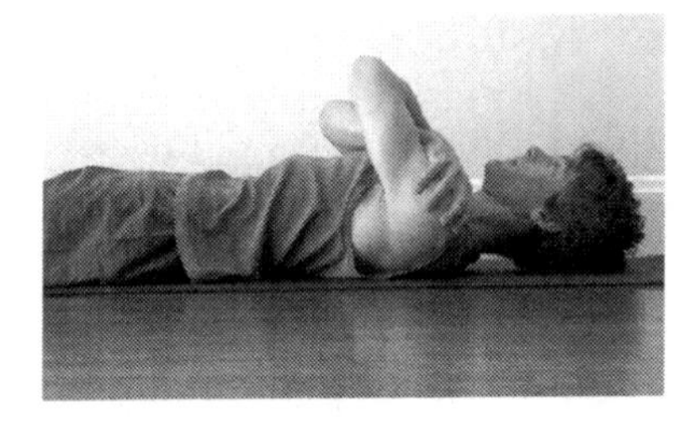

- The sub occipital muscles connect the base of the skull to the top of the spine and are the only muscles in the body with an energetic connection to the eyes. They tend to be chronically short.
- Lie flat on your back and bring a small natural arch to your lower back. The legs should be straight; you can put a blanket under the knees if there is any strain on the lower back.
- Raise your arms to the sky, pulling your shoulder blades away from the floor. Try to let the upper spine settle onto the ground. Grasp each shoulder with the opposite hand.
- Lengthen the back of the neck as much as you can without closing off or creating discomfort at the front of the throat.
- Stay for three minutes to start, and try to build up to five minutes.

12. Fingers in the direction of the toes

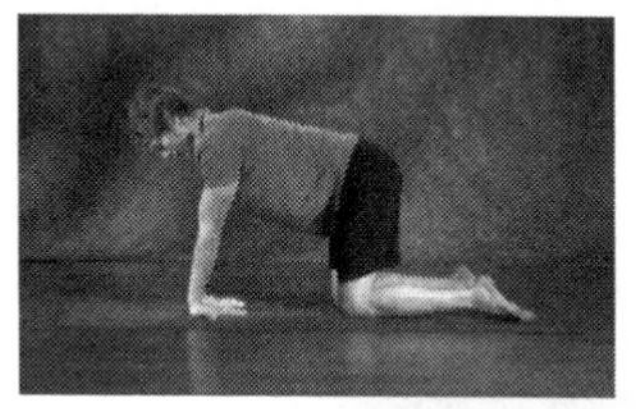

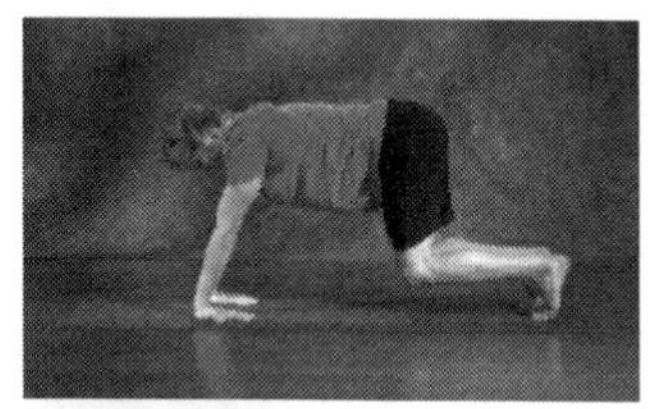

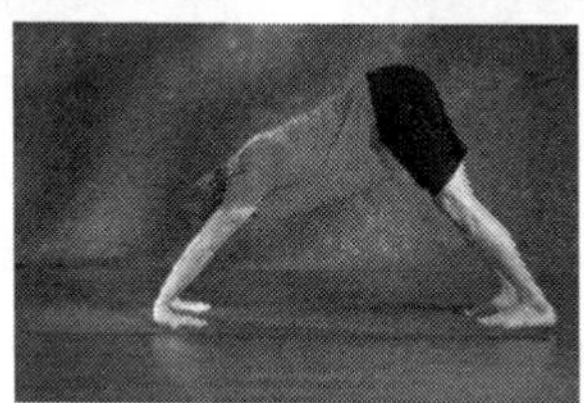

- Start on your hands and knees and turn your hand around bringing your fingers in the direction of your toes. Do you best to get the middle finger in line with the center of the kneecap.
- Stretch the hips back a little. This might be very intense.
- If it is not too bad, lift the knees one inch off of the floor.
- If all is good, go to downward dog.
- Everything should be easy.

VII- The Cactus Group

1. Cactus at the Wall

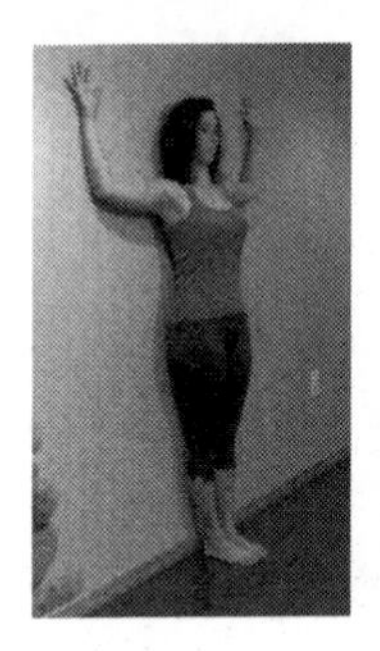
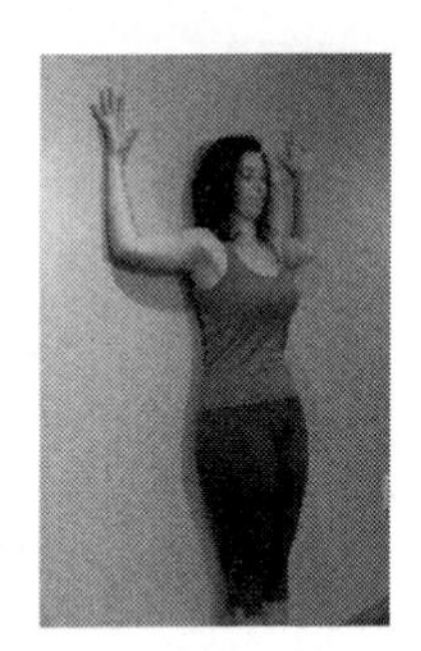

- Stand with your back to a wall. Place your feet about six inches away from the wall. Relax your knees.
- Bring your arms out to the side and press everything to the wall (except for the neck and low back), focusing on the middle of your back.
- Slowly bend the elbows bringing your hands up to a right angle with your arms. Make sure everything remains on the wall. Move very slowly.
- If the arms come to a right angle, move the elbows up the wall, keeping everything connected.

2. Cactus on the Back

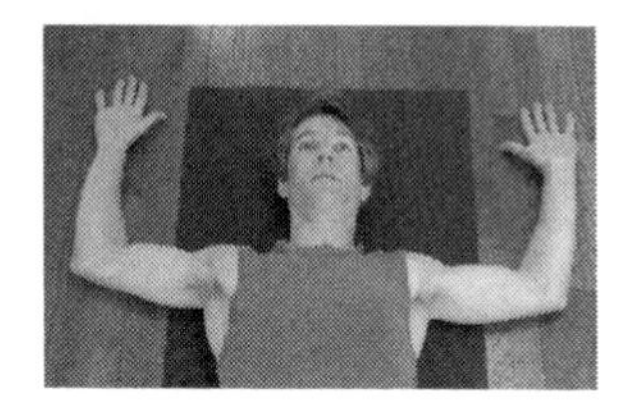

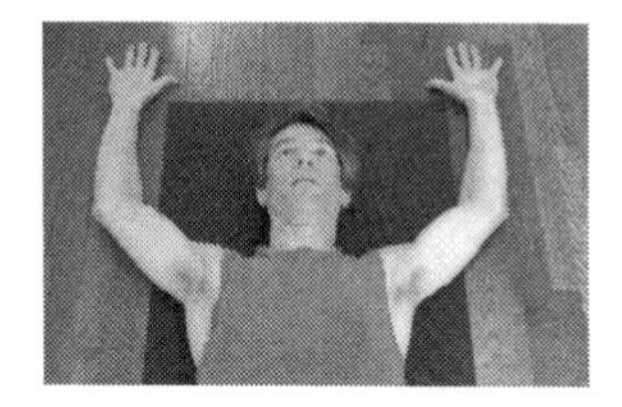

This falls somewhere between a release and a stretch and is not nearly as benign as some of these explorations. In fact, this can be very intense, though you won't be doing much.

- Lie flat on your back. If it is not comfortable to lie with the legs straight, roll up a blanket and place it under the knees. This will release the hamstrings and reduce the strain on the lower back.
- Bring your arms out to the side and bend your elbows to form a right angle with the arms.
- Lengthen the back of the neck and allow the spine to soften toward the floor. The lower back and neck should each have a gentle arch, but ideally the rest of the spine should have contact with the floor. Move very slowly.
- Once you get your spine into a good place, bring your awareness to the forearms, wrists and hands. Try to open the hands, extending the wrists and the fingers. Move very slowly.

- Once you get the arm to a good place return to the spine. Go back and forth between the two and allow the back of the body to lengthen, soften, and release.

3. **Cactus on the Belly**

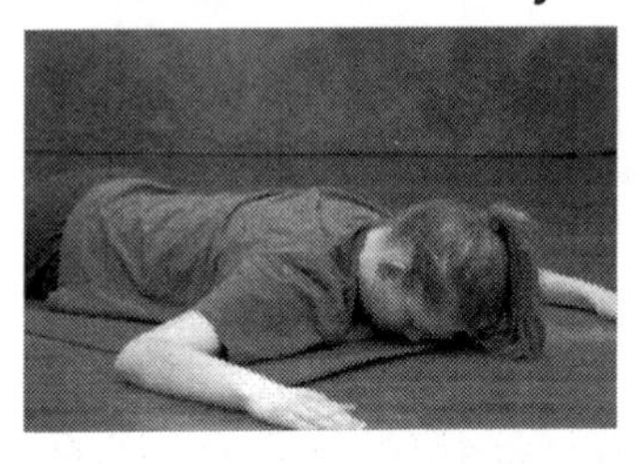

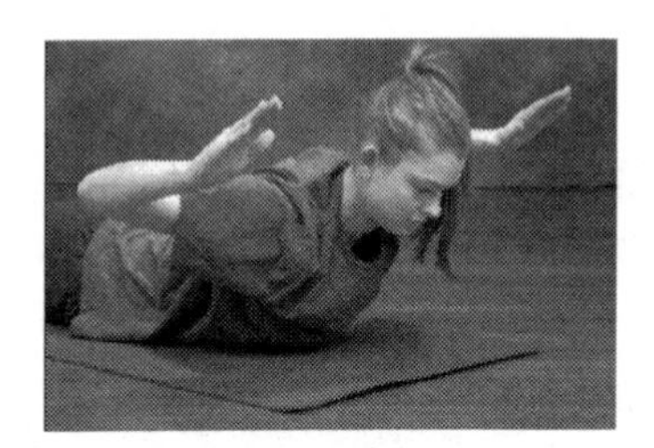

- Lie flat on your belly.
- Bring your arms out to the side and bend your elbows to form a right angle with the arms.
- Lengthen the back of the neck.
- Once you get your spine into a good place, bring your awareness to the forearms, wrists and hands. Everything is balanced before you lift up, the forearms wrists and fingers are all balanced between extension and flexion.
- Lift the head neck and chest up off of the floor. Notice the difficulty in maintaining the balance in the different parts of the arm.

VII. Releases

1. Constructive Rest (CRP)

CONSTRUCTIVE REST POSITION (CRP)

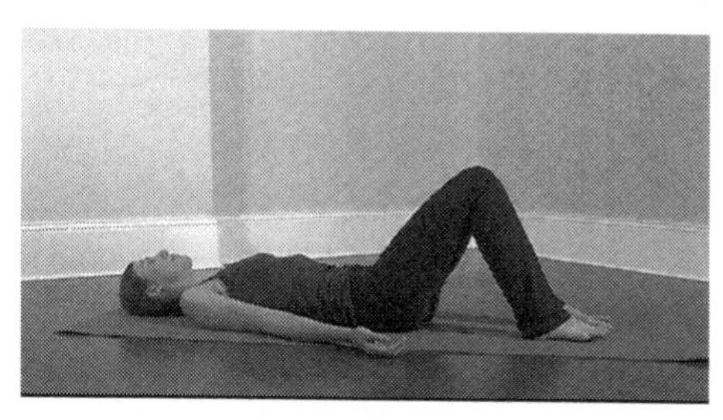

This is the main psoas release that we work with. It is a gravitational release of the psoas that allows the force of gravity to have its way with the contents of the trunk and the deep core.

- Lie on your back with your knees bent and your heels situated 12 to 16 inches away from your pelvis, in line with your sit bones.
- Tie a belt around the middle of the thighs. You want to be able to let go here and not have to think too much about the position of your legs.
- Then do nothing. Discomfort arises from conditioned muscular patterns. Try not to shift or move when unpleasant sensations arise.

- You are hoping to feel sensations that you can sit with, and if possible, allow it to pass.
- Try to do this for 30 minutes a day. If you have time, longer sessions are advisable or twice a day.

But you are not here to suffer. If sensations come up and you feel that you have to move, feel free to move, then come back to where you were and try again. It's possible that you'll do this exercise and not feel anything; it will still be good for you.

2. Foot on a Block

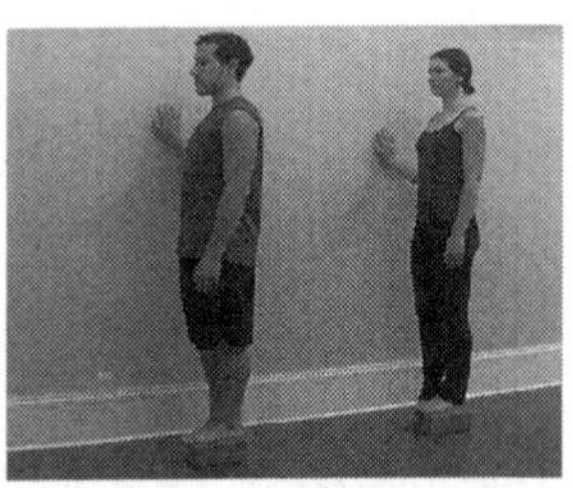

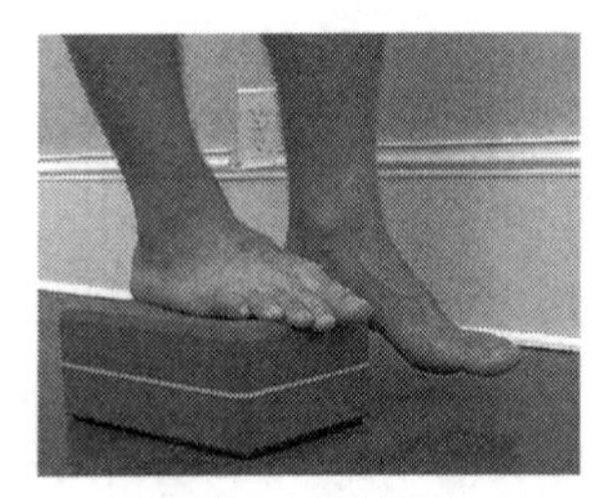

This is another gravitational release of the psoas. This exercise is not limited to your house. If you have hip or groin pain when walking, feel free to stop at every corner and dangle one foot off of the curb while holding on to a lamp post.

- Place a block eight to ten inches from a wall.

- Step the left foot up on the block, allowing the right foot to hang down between the block and the wall. Place your right arm on the wall to help you stabilize the upper body.
- Keep the hips level and rotate the inner thighs back and apart—stick out your butt a bit, and feel like you can let the leg go from the base of the rib cage, the top of the psoas.
- Once you are comfortable with the leg hanging out of the hip, you can move the leg half an inch forward and back as slowly and steadily as possible. Half an inch is a very short distance.
- Let the leg dangle this way for 30 seconds or until the standing hip has done enough.
- Switch sides and tune in to which side is tighter. Do the second side for the same length of time that you did on the first side.
- Repeat for a second time on the tighter side.

3. Tight Hip Release

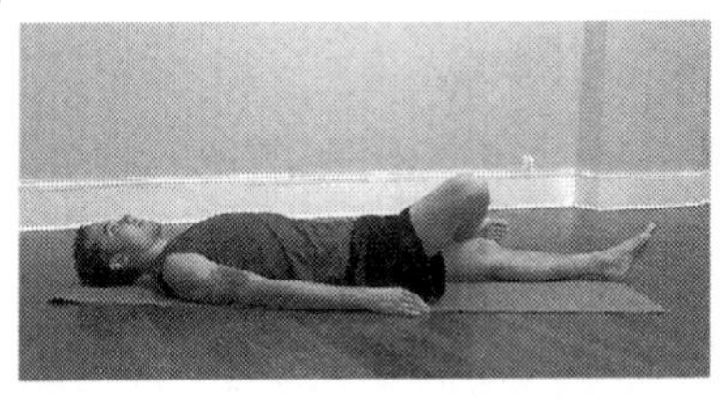

This is meant as a passive release for extremely tight hips. If your knee is higher than a 45-degree angle from the floor when you assume this position, this exercise is for you.

- Lie on your back with the legs straight out on the floor. Stabilize the trunk and bring the right foot as high up on the left thigh as possible.
- Allow the right knee to release toward the floor, keeping the trunk stable the entire time.
- Try to let the release come from both the inner and outer thigh as gravity takes the leg toward the floor.
- Stay for five minutes on each side if possible.

4. Block Lunges

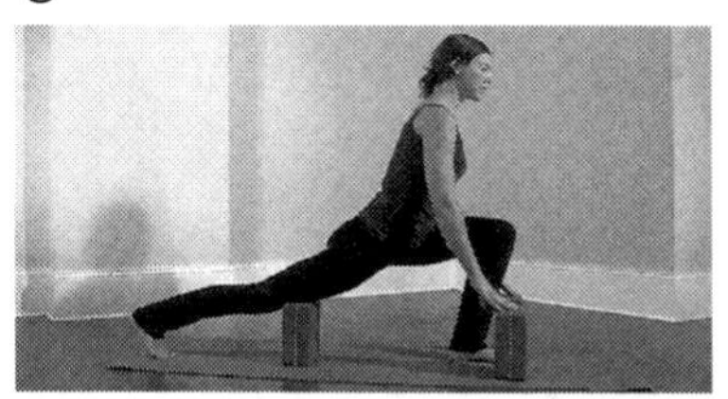

This is a release of both the quadriceps and the psoas. Sometimes the quadriceps muscles are so tight, there is no getting to the psoas until we release the quads a bit. You'll need three blocks for this.

- Positioned on your hands and knees or in Downward Facing Dog, step the right foot forward in between your hands. Two blocks will be for your hands by the front foot.
- Place the third block underneath the quadriceps muscle just above the knee, at the base of the thigh.
- Tuck the back toes and let the weight of the body fall onto the block. Do your best to keep the heel of the back foot pointing straight up toward the ceiling.
- The front leg and hip should not be under any strain. Feel free to make adjustments, turning the foot out or stepping the foot wider.
- You need to stay for 90 seconds to get the full benefits of this pose.

5. Ankle to Knee Backwards

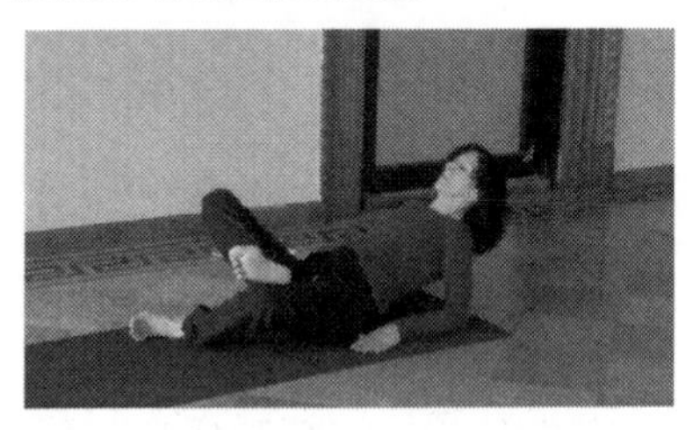

This exercise is meant to release your piriformis muscle but often involves intense sensation in the quadriceps tendon or the IT band.

- In a seated position, bend your knees and try to stack your shins on top of one another. Your right foot should be on your left knee and your right knee should hover or lay flat above your left foot. If your left knee is higher than twelve inches off of the ground or seems like it can't even get into such a position extend your left knee straight. If you do stack your shins, you should see an even triangle of space between your pelvis and you shins.
- You can loosely belt the legs in a way that doesn't pull them closer to each other but also won't let them separate any further.
- Begin to lean backwards slowly keeping an arch in your lower back. You have to keep the natural arch of the back even if you can only go a few inches. You can go down as far as your

forearms, trying to relax and allow the right inner and outer thigh to release passively with each breath.

6. Frog Belly

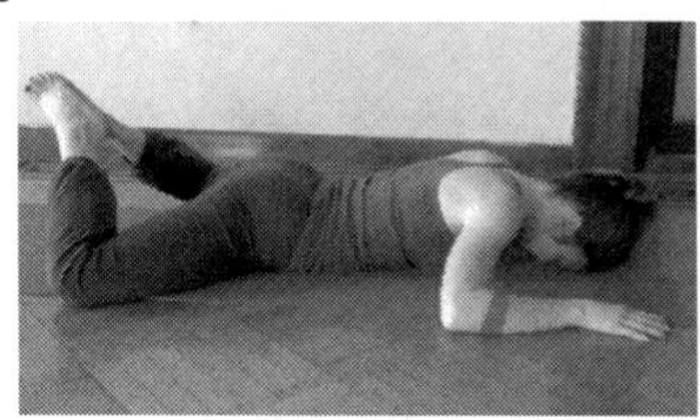

This is another piriformis release. In letting the piriformis at the back relax, muscles at the front of the thigh often complain. Do your best to let it go.

- Lay on your stomach. Bend your knees wide out to the side, bringing the soles of the feet together in mid-air. They will likely be high off the floor.
- The top of the pelvis should be on the floor determining the height of the feet.
- Relax. Draw the knees as wide as possible and allow the feet to separate slightly can deepen this pose.
  Relax. Let gravity work on your feet while you keep the pelvis grounded.

7. Ankle over knee at wall

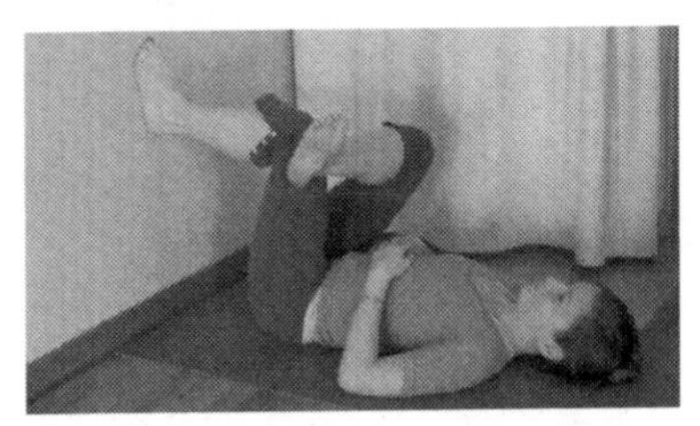

- Lay on your back with your pelvis about a foot or a foot and a half from the wall.
- Cross the right ankle over the left knee and bring the left foot to the wall at the height of your hip. You might need to adjust the distance between the pelvis and the wall to get the correct tension.
- Let your right knee open passively. Stay for up to ten or even fifteen minutes.

8. Differentiating Leg From Trunk

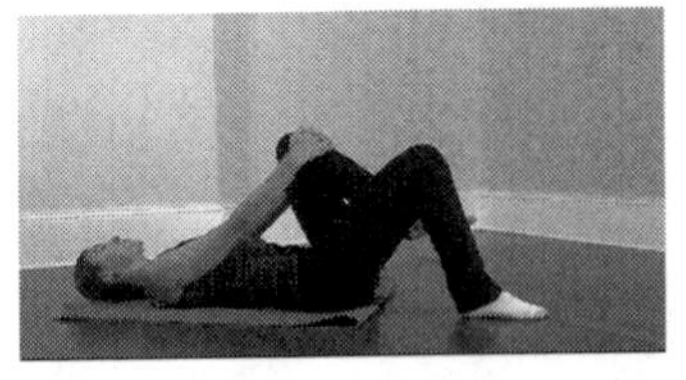

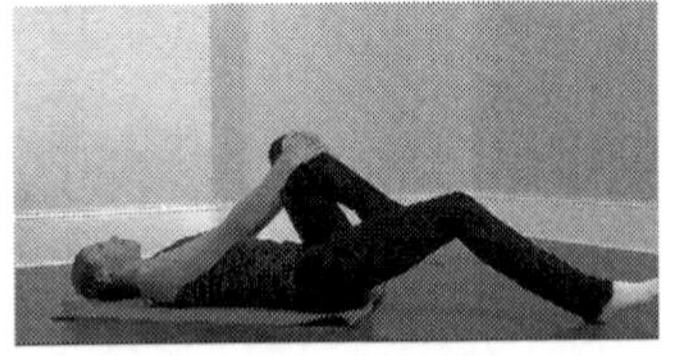

- Bend the left knee and interlace your fingers at the top of the shin. Hold the leg out at arm's length. Extend the other leg. Pay attention to the hip socket—only move your leg, not the pelvis.
- Bring tone to the pelvic floor and the low belly and do your best to stabilize the trunk.
- Extend the right leg out slowly. It doesn't have to extend completely.

- Slowly lift the right knee up, drawing the heel toward the hip and keeping the left heel on the floor with the foot flexed.
- Maintaining a stable trunk, extend the right leg out again.
- Repeat ten times on each side if possible. Feel free to start with as few as three times.

9. Releasing Arms

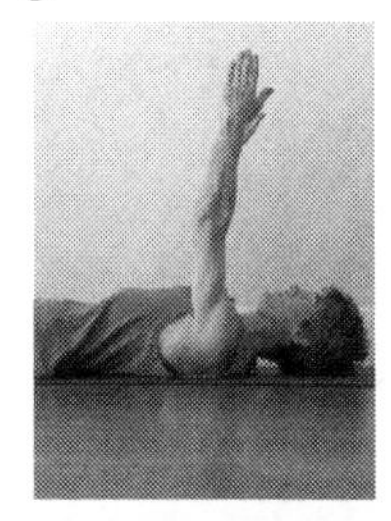
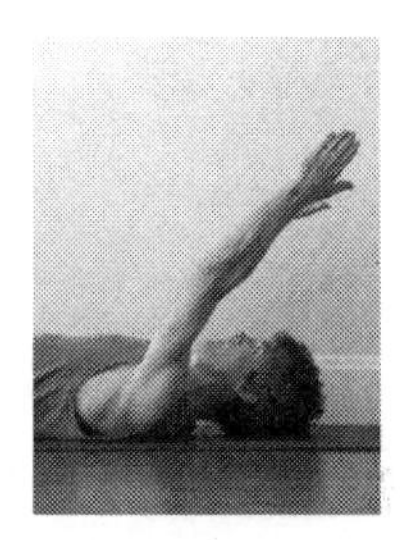

This exercise works on the ability to articulate the arms separately from the trunk.

- Lie flat on your back and bring your arms up, with the fingers pointing toward the ceiling.
- Begin to lower the arms over head, trying to keep the rib cage and spine from moving.
- Focus on keeping the trunk still. Stop lowering the arms once the trunk moves.
- The eyes and head can follow the arms in movement. As you go deeper the arms should stay parallel and the elbows shouldn't

bend.

1(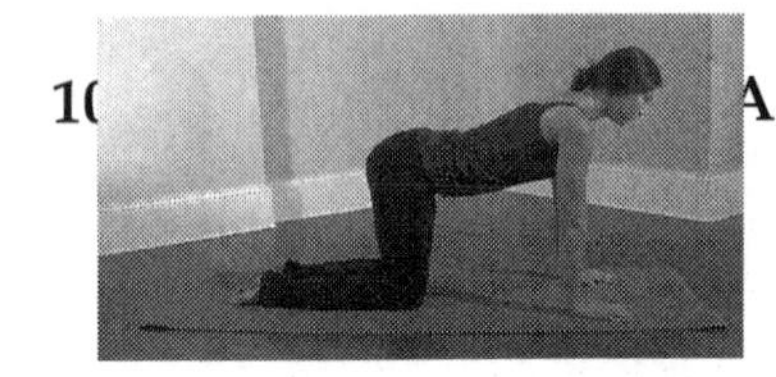 **Anc** 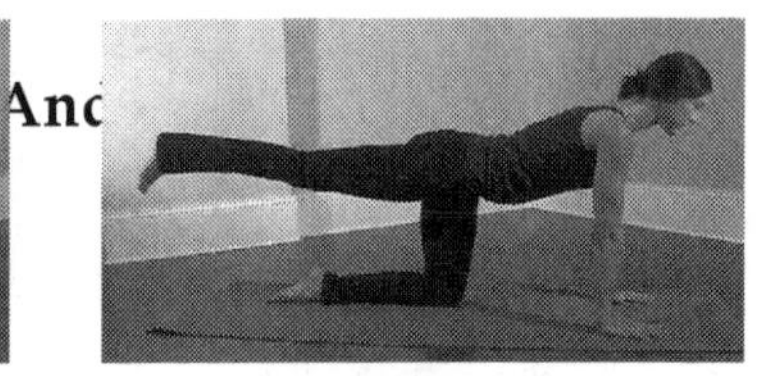

This exercise explores the ability of the leg to separate from the pelvis and the spine.

- Start on your hands and knees with the hips over the knees and the wrists underneath the shoulders.
- Bring gentle tone to the pelvic floor and the lower belly and try to extend your right leg back, bringing the leg level with the trunk.
- Keep your awareness on the lower back and the pelvis stabilizing the trunk to release the leg.
- As always, these are experiential exercises where you try to get a feeling for what the body is doing. The tighter psoas will be the side that can't move without pulling the pelvis and the spine with it.

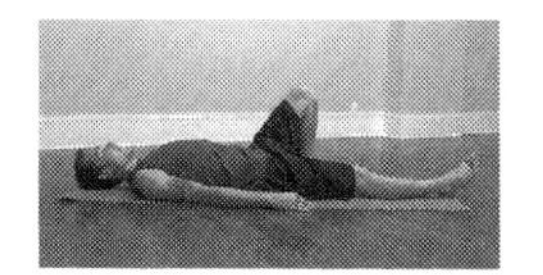 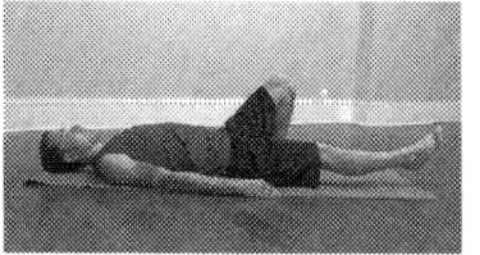 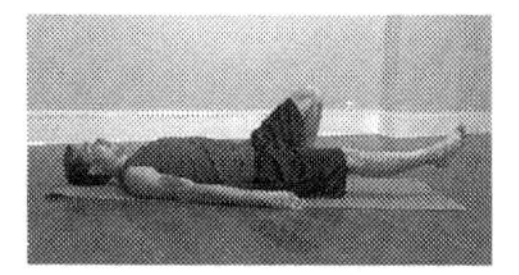

The following exercise works the psoas more than most of these explorations. Proceed slowly, and don't overdo it in the beginning.

- Begin in constructive rest. Extend the right leg straight out.
- Press the left foot down into the floor to help the right leg lift up two inches.
- Lift the right leg three or four inches higher, and then lower it back to two inches off the floor.
- Repeat five times if possible, keeping the pelvis and spine stable. The only thing working is the leg.
- Switch sides.

Once you are comfortable taking the leg up and down, begin again by pressing the opposite foot into the floor. One variation is to move the leg from side to side, and another is to move the leg on a diagonal, staying within a three- or four-inch range of motion.

Note: Three inches is a very short distance.

12. Reclining Cobbler's Pose

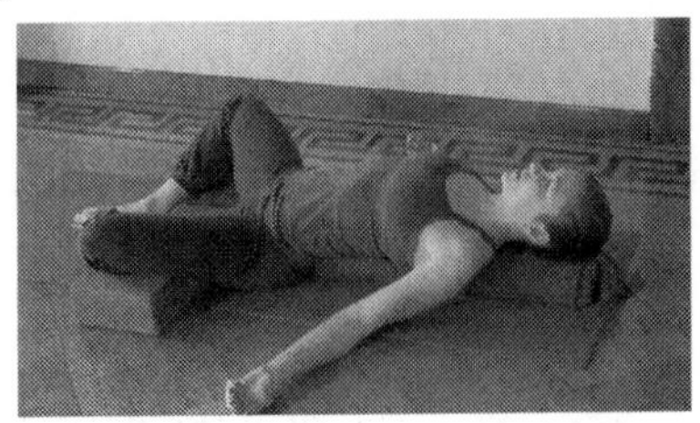

- Lay flat on your back with a blanket or towel rolled up, lengthwise under your spine. You could also place pillows under you. Your torso and head should feel supported. Make sure the head is extending with the spine and not dropping back.
- Bring the soles of the feet together as close to the hips as possible.
- Keeping the soles of the feet together, let the knees fall open to the side.
- Support the outer leg with blocks or blankets or pillows under the thighs.
- Let everything go as long as you feel supported in the shape.
- This puts the piriformis at rest, not allowing it to do anything.
- Try to stay for 10 – 20 minutes

13. Soft Ball Under Sacrum And/Or Neck

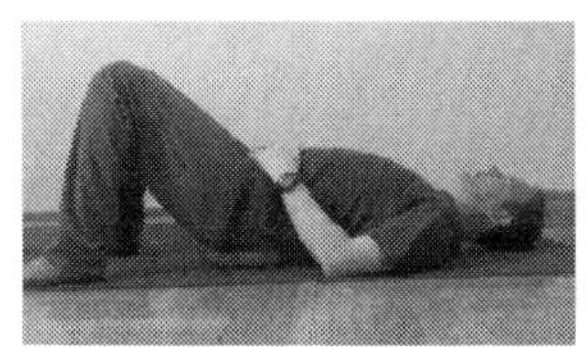
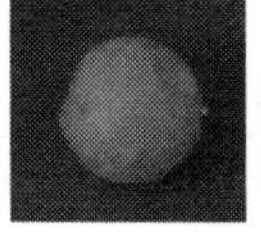
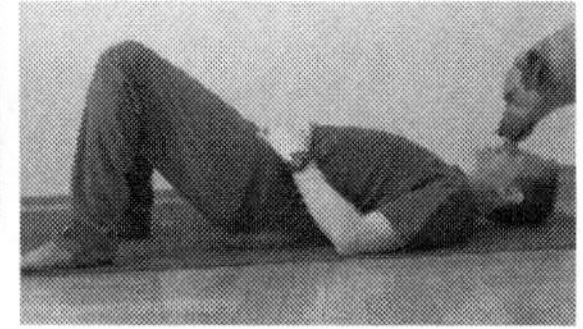

- You need a very soft and pliable ball for this exercise.
- Place the ball under your sacrum and relax onto it.
- You can roll around a little but basically just try to stay still.
- After a few minutes (up to 15) deflate the ball a little bit and move it to the base of the head. Not under the neck, but at the place where the spine meet the cranium.
- Chill.

14. Orange Thing

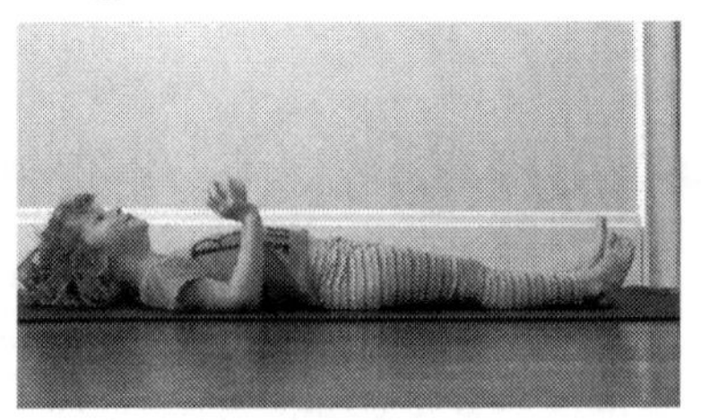

- This is more for fun than anything else. Look at yourself in a mirror before and after you have done one side and see if notice a difference.
- Lay flat on your back with an orange or a ball of similar size sitting by your right hip.
- Roll the orange slowly back and forth from the heel of your palm to the fingertips.
- Pick up the orange and hold it in your open palm with the elbow on the floor and the palm facing the ceiling.
- Balance the orange on your palm for two or three minutes before stopping.

VIII. Acknowledgements

I have learned from so many people both in person and in print. Here is a short list of those who influenced this book:

Therese Bertherat, Genny Kapuler, Bonnie Bainbridge Cohen, Irene Dowd, John Friend, Sandra Jamrog, Bessel van der Kolk, Liz Koch, Peter Levine, Tom Myers, Jenny Otto, Ida Rolf, Lulu Sweigard.

Thanks as well to artists and Models:

Maya Brand

Molly Fitzsimons

Caitlin FitzGordon

Ida FitzGordon

Heather Greer

Beth Hyde

Jesse Kaminash

Chris Marx

David Martinez

Christopher Moore

Raina Passo

Special thanks to Katie Malachuk.

Made in the USA
San Bernardino, CA
19 November 2016